Lynda AOUDIA

Breast MRI

Lynda AOUDIA

Breast MRI

ScienciaScripts

Imprint
Any brand names and product names mentioned in this book are subject to trademark, brand or patent protection and are trademarks or registered trademarks of their respective holders. The use of brand names, product names, common names, trade names, product descriptions etc. even without a particular marking in this work is in no way to be construed to mean that such names may be regarded as unrestricted in respect of trademark and brand protection legislation and could thus be used by anyone.

Cover image: www.ingimage.com

This book is a translation from the original published under ISBN 978-620-3-44483-4.

Publisher:
Sciencia Scripts
is a trademark of
Dodo Books Indian Ocean Ltd. and OmniScriptum S.R.L publishing group

120 High Road, East Finchley, London, N2 9ED, United Kingdom
Str. Armeneasca 28/1, office 1, Chisinau MD-2012, Republic of Moldova, Europe
Managing Directors: Ieva Konstantinova, Victoria Ursu
info@omniscriptum.com

Printed at: see last page
ISBN: 978-620-8-57051-4

Contents

Foreword

Breast MRI is now an essential part of the breast assessment, and is sufficiently sensitive to detect breast lesions smaller than 3 mm. It has become the preferred screening test for women at high risk of breast cancer.

The problem with breast MRI is that it has a long learning curve, is a complex method, has many pitfalls and requires experience.

The aim of this educational book is to explain and describe the different morphological and kinetic signs of breast lesions on MRI, in order to make our interpretation as accurate as possible and reduce diagnostic errors.

Compliance with the indications, optimisation of acquisition protocols and knowledge of the various breast MRI semiological signs will ensure correct interpretation and minimise diagnostic errors.

Consistent and explicit diagrams are used throughout the book to describe the morphological and kinetic signs of breast lesions:

- definition of MRI sign ;
- demonstrative scheme ;
- example: MRI images and interpretation.

This book aims to clarify and speed up the clinical application of breast MRI, so that doctors can make the most accurate and reliable diagnosis.

Professor Lynda AOUDIA

Introduction

Breast imaging began with mammography, which can detect cancers with a sensitivity of 70-90% in women aged over 50 [1,6]. Mammography has good spatial resolution and high contrast resolution, enabling it to detect certain abnormalities such as microcalcifications. However, its sensitivity is much lower in patients with dense breasts, ranging from 30% to 48% depending on the series [7, 8]. Ultrasound is a very useful examination in dense breasts, in order to detect and characterise isodense lesions in glandular tissue on mammography. Glandular tissue is more hyperechoic than fat, and cancerous lesions are easier to see as they are usually hypoechoic. Ultrasound can also distinguish between simple benign cysts and solid masses. However, ultrasound cannot reliably visualise microcalcifications. Colour Doppler detects intratumoral vascularisation. It can identify whether hypoechoic lesions are cystic or solid. The presence of vascularisation within the echogenic portion makes it possible to distinguish a tissue lesion from intracystic debris. Doppler, on the other hand, allows only a limited study of tumour vascularisation. According to the work of Folkman, tumour angiogenesis plays a key role in cancer growth [9, 10]. The detection of neoangiogenesis is a highly sensitive indicator of the presence of a tumour.

MRI (Magnetic Resonance Imaging) of the breast is increasingly used in breast assessment. MRI is a non-invasive, non-irradiating technique that can detect lesions with abnormally developed microcirculation compared with adjacent tissues, giving it very high sensitivity, ranging from 85% to 100% [11-14]. Microcirculatory differences are detected by comparing the enhancement of lesions and adjacent fibroglandular tissue after injection of contrast medium. This difference in enhancement corresponds to a difference in the concentration of contrast agent in the lesions compared with normal breast tissue. However, this technique generates a certain number of false positives, due to the number of benign lesions which also show a more developed microcirculation than the surrounding fibroglandular tissue, thus reducing its specificity (65-80%) [1114]. Compliance with the indications, optimisation of the acquisition protocol, good knowledge of the various MRI semiological signs and integration of its interpretation into the overall breast assessment are the guarantees of the diagnostic value of this examination for patient management.

1. Indications for breast MRI

There are a number of indications for which breast MRI is expected to add diagnostic value. Breast MRI is currently validated for screening for breast cancer in women at very high genetic risk (BRCA1 and 2 gene mutations, other genetic mutations) or for diagnosis, often performed as a complement to mammography-ultrasound. There are other indications, such as the assessment of breast cancer extension, dense breasts or subtle lesions on conventional imaging [15]. This examination is recommended in the following cases

1.1. Screening women at high risk of breast cancer

Several genetic mutations predispose to a high risk of breast or ovarian cancer, such as BRCA1, BRCA2, p53 mutation (Li-Fraumeni syndrome), PTEN (Cowden's disease) and STK11 (Peutz-Jeghers syndrome). In women with a BRCA1 mutation, the cumulative absolute lifetime risk of developing breast cancer is over 80% [16]. According to European recommendations, screening MRI should be performed from the age of 30. However, in some cases, screening MRI may be started before the age of 30: between the ages of 25 and 29 for patients with a BRCA1 or BRCA2 mutation; from the age of 20 for patients with a p53 mutation. The sensitivity of MRI for detecting breast cancer in this at-risk population was 71% to 100% depending on the series, compared with 13% to 40% for mammography [17-24]. The difference in sensitivity between MRI and mammography can be explained by the lower sensitivity of mammography in dense breasts [25]. On the basis of these results, screening MRI for women at high risk of breast cancer was considered. This technique makes it possible to detect cancers at an early stage and reduce the risk of lymph node extension. Some studies have reported that 19% of patients screened by MRI had lymph node involvement, compared with 50% of patients not screened by MRI [26, 27].

1.2. Characterisation of ambiguous anomalies on conventional imaging when biopsy is not possible

MRI is increasingly prescribed to try to characterise images that are ambiguous on conventional imaging. However, it is preferable to perform a biopsy for lesions that are accessible and classified as BIRADS 4 or 5. MRI may be indicated in the following cases: subtle image not biopsiable on mammography and not visible on ultrasound, suspicious mammographic image visible on a single incidence, focal asymmetries of density, multiple masses suspicious on ultrasound, differential diagnosis of a complicated cyst [11].

1.3. Search for an occult primary cancer in a metastasis work-up

In patients with axillary lymph node metastases, or metastases suggestive of primary breast cancer, these represent 1% of breast cancers [28, 29]. MRI can detect occult primary cancer in 61% of patients [30-32]. MRI is indicated in cases of suspected breast metastases where clinical examination and conventional imaging are negative.

1.4. Inflammatory breast cancer

The risk of carcinomatous mastitis is lower than that of inflammatory or infectious mastitis. Breast MRI is indicated if inflammatory symptoms persist after appropriate medical treatment (anti-inflammatory drugs ± antibiotics) for 15 days. The aim of MRI is to differentiate carcinomatous mastitis by looking for the presence of a mass, located posteriorly, with suspicious enhancement.

1.5. Local extension assessment of breast cancer

The therapeutic strategy for breast cancer is based on the most accurate assessment possible of its location, size (particularly in dense breasts, infiltrating lobular carcinoma and ductal carcinoma in situ) and extension. The recognised advantage of MRI is that it allows a more reliable assessment of the pre-therapeutic extension of breast cancer than mammography and ultrasound [33, 34]. MRI is better at assessing the size of the cancer and local spread. It is also more effective in detecting multifocality (same quadrant), multicentricity (different quadrants) or bilaterality. MRI can also be used to assess cutaneomuscular extension.

To date, no study has really assessed the impact of breast MRI extension assessment on survival. Furthermore, systematic preoperative breast MRI does not reduce the rate of repeat surgery. Some studies have therefore reported that systematic breast MRI as part of the preoperative breast cancer extension assessment is not currently recommended [35, 36].

MRI should not delay treatment (the delay before treatment should not exceed one month).

1.6. Evaluation of response to neoadjuvant chemotherapy

Neoadjuvant chemotherapy is usually indicated in two clinical situations:

- inoperable breast cancers at initial diagnosis ;
- operable breast cancers (stages IIa, IIb, IIIa) for which conservative surgery

is not immediately accessible.

An initial MRI should be carried out as a reference prior to chemotherapy, to enable an initial extension assessment to be carried out, specifying the number of lesions, whether single or multiple, and assessing skin and muscle extension.

Intermediate MRI after the second course of neoadjuvant chemotherapy (C2) is used to detect non-responders so that treatment can be changed [37]. MRI at C2 can also be used to detect patients who have responded to treatment and who need to have a clip placed in the residual tumour in order to visualise the tumour bed during preoperative positioning.

End-of-treatment MRI is performed within two weeks of the end of chemotherapy and during the week before surgery. This mammary MRI is used to guide the surgical procedure, by assessing the residual tumour volume, differentiating concentric tumour melts after chemotherapy (possible lumpectomy) from tumour melts with multiple foci (mastectomy), and detecting insufficient response for conservative treatment (lesion

• 3 cm after chemotherapy). A number of studies have assessed tumour volume after chemotherapy using breast MRI, and have reported that MRI is clearly superior to clinical examination, mammography and ultrasound [38-42].

1.7. Recurrence of treated breast cancer

The risk of recurrence after conservative treatment is around 0.5% per year and approximately 5% at 15 years [43, 44]. Most recurrences are detected by conventional imaging and confirmed histologically by biopsy.

However, analysis of the surgical site is sometimes difficult with conventional imaging. MRI has a high sensitivity, estimated at between 90% and 100% for detecting local recurrence [45-47].

1.8. Monitoring silicone-containing prostheses

The fitting of a breast prosthesis for aesthetic purposes or in the case of reconstruction after breast cancer surgery. Most breast implants are made of silicone only (single-lumen implant) or are combined with physiological saline (double-lumen implant). It is important to know the type of implant so that the radiologist can optimise the breast MRI protocol. The risk of rupture of the latest generation prosthesis is around 5% at five years [48-50]. MRI is the most effective test for assessing prosthesis integrity compared with mammography and ultrasound [51]. MRI can also reveal intra- and extracapsular ruptures and assess the extent of silicone leakage in the breast.

Breast MRI is highly sensitive for detecting tumour recurrence in breast prostheses [51].

1.9. Breast discharge

In the case of unipore breast discharge, conventional imaging and cytological analysis of the discharge are necessary, as it may be secondary to a malignant or high-risk lesion. MRI would be useful to help identify an intraductal lesion, especially if it is distal and difficult to identify on galactography.

1.10. Male breast cancer

Male breast cancer is rare, accounting for 1% of breast cancers [52]. MRI would be useful in assessing tumour extension to the pectoral muscle [53]. Breast MRI may also be indicated for screening men with a proven BRCA 2 genetic mutation, after multidisciplinary consultation, and for monitoring the efficacy of neoadjuvant chemotherapy.

CHAPTER 2

2. Contraindications of MRI

Before undergoing an MRI scan, there are a number of contraindications to be considered:

2.1. Absolute contraindications

Absolute contraindications must always be respected, without the slightest exception.

Any metallic body on the patient that is likely to move under the effect of the MRI magnetic field may constitute an absolute contraindication, and a real MRI hazard.

- Patient with a pacemaker.
- Old-generation heart valves.
- Old-generation ferromagnetic vascular surgical clips for treating endocranial aneurysms.
- Neurosimulators, cochlear implants, automated injection devices such as insulin pumps, and more generally any non-removable electronic medical equipment.
- Ocular metallic foreign body: a control X-ray is then necessary to determine whether this is an absolute or relative contraindication.

2.2. Relative contraindications

Contraindications are said to be relative when it is possible, under certain conditions.

In all these cases, the radiologist assesses the MRI benefit/risk ratio.

2.2.1. Relative contraindication linked to the device

- For claustrophobic patients, open-field MRI is sometimes a solution.

2.2.2. Relative contraindications linked to the magnetic field

- Various metallic implants: this depends on the position of the foreign body in relation to the area examined by medical imaging.
- Transdermal patch with risk of local burning.
- Stent: after a stent has been inserted, it is preferable to wait 8 to 12 weeks to avoid any MRI risks. After this time, the stent is integrated into the tissue so that it poses no risk to the patient. MRI can normally be performed despite the presence of a cardiac stent.
- Pregnancy: the precautionary principle means that MRI should be avoided during the first 4 months of pregnancy. If the examination cannot wait until after the birth, the radiologist will assess the benefit/risk ratio.

CHAPTER 3

3. Breast MRI technique

3.1. Equipment

3.1.1. Magnetic field

Magnetic field strength affects acquisition time and image quality. The higher the magnetic field strength, the better the image resolution and the shorter the sequences. Most teams work with magnetic fields of 1.5 tesla (T).

3.1.2. Antennas

Breast MRI must be performed using dedicated breast antennas that follow the shape of the breasts (fig. 1). The use of parallel imaging improves the performance of these antennas, increasing the area covered, signal uniformity, and temporal and spatial resolution [15]. The breasts must be well positioned in the antenna, with the nipple at the zenith, integrating the entire breast into the antenna and avoiding folds (fig. 2).

The breast should not be compressed too much. Compression is used to support the breasts to prevent them moving in the antenna. Excessive compression of the breast can falsely reduce the size of lesions and thus change the TNM classification [54]. Compression can also reduce the amplitude of enhancement and modify the enhancement curve (fig. 3).

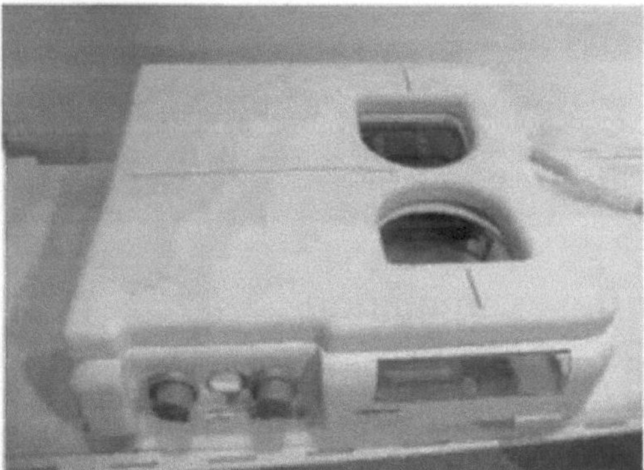

Fig. 1. breast antenna.

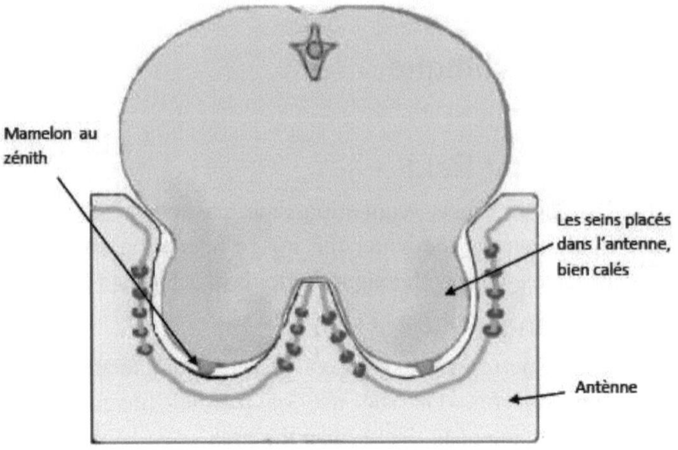

Nipple at the Antènne zenith
The breasts placed in the antenna, well supported
Fig. 2 Position of the breasts in the anterior.

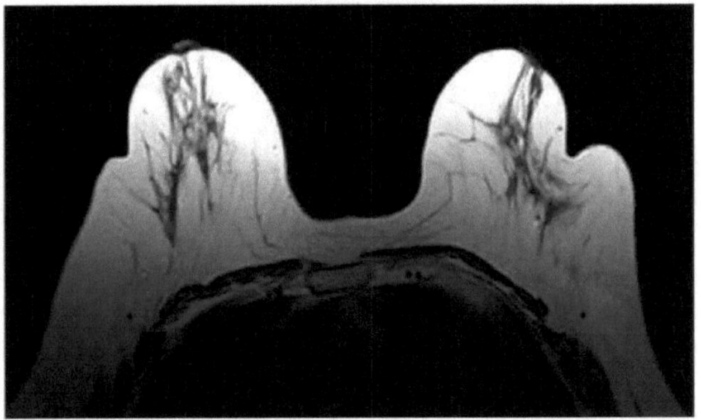

Fig. 3: Compression defect. T2-weighted sequence

3.2. Time of the examination

The timing of the examination is essential for a better interpretation of breast MRI. The second part of the cycle should be avoided, when physiological glandular enhancement is most marked. It is minimal in the 2nd week of the menstrual cycle in patients who are genitally active. Outside this period, there may be diffuse non-specific contrast, but also focal contrast, which may lead to misinterpretation (fig. 4). Glandular enhancement is increased by hormone replacement therapy in post-menopausal women, with up to 50% of women showing non-specific enhancement. A 3-month stop in the event of an uninterpretable examination in post-menopausal women.

For postoperative MRI, a minimum delay of one month should be observed in order to limit enhancement secondary to inflammatory phenomena; the optimum time for performing breast MRI is at least six months after the end of treatment [55-57].

Percutaneous microbiopsies do not generally affect the interpretation of contrast-enhanced MRI. However, the topography, date of biopsies and results, if available, should always be mentioned. Oral contraception also has no impact on the use of breast MRI.

3.3. Settling the patient

A venous access with a long tube is put in place. The patient is then placed in the procubitus position, with her arms over her head as comfortably as possible, to ensure the immobility required for the examination. The breasts placed in the antenna must be well supported; if necessary, a foam pad can be used to prevent the small breasts from moving in the antenna (fig. 5).

3.4. Injection of contrast medium

Breast MRI highlights intratumoral neoangiogenesis through the injection of contrast, enabling lesions to be detected [11]. The contrast agent used is gadolinium chelate. The dose injected 0.1 mmol/kg body weight. The injection rate should be 2 to 3 ml per second. The injection of the contrast product is followed by an injection of 20 ml of physiological saline at the same rate to avoid stagnation of the contrast product in the tubing.

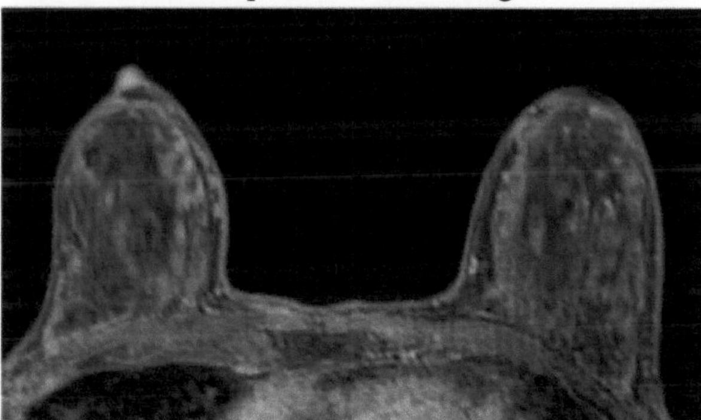

Fig. 4: Physiological glandular enhancement. Subtracted sequence injected

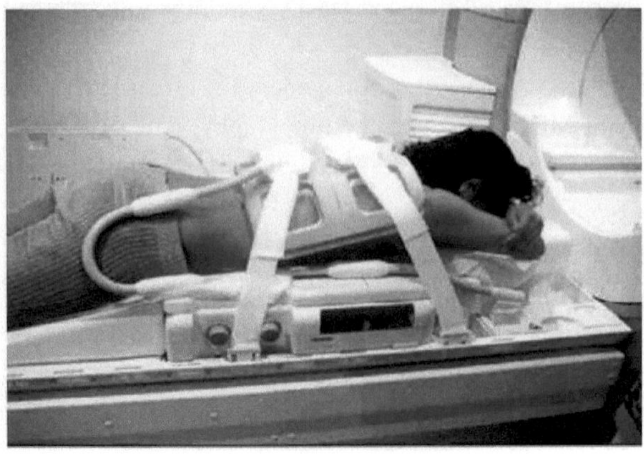

Fig. 5: Patient settles in.

3.5. Breast MRI protocols

3.5.1. Acquisition plan

The fields of view must be wide enough to analyse both breasts, both nipple-areolar plates (NAPs), the axillary hollows and the chest wall [11, 58].
Acquisition in the axial plane is the most frequently used. This acquisition plane makes it possible to carry out dynamic sequences of the breasts in 1 minute. The advantages of the axial plane are that the entirety of both breasts can be analysed comparatively, which makes it easier to detect abnormal contrast, and also allows analysis of the PAM, the axillary fossae and the chest wall [58]. Cardiorespiratory artefacts degrade the quality of acquisitions. Phase encoding from right to left instead of anteroposterior reduces these artefacts.
Acquisition in the sagittal plane makes it possible to reduce the field of view. This improves image resolution and the quality of fat suppression techniques [11]. Finally, sagittal acquisition also allows better analysis of physiological glandular enhancement, which facilitates anatomical study. Nevertheless, the study of both breasts with the axillary hollows requires a large number of slices, which prolongs the examination time [58].
Coronal acquisition reduces cardiac artefacts. However, this plane is often degraded by respiratory and flow artefacts. This acquisition plane also requires a large number of slices to be able to analyse the entire breast from the chest wall to the PAM [58].

3.5.2. Cutting thickness

The slice thickness must be thin, less than or equal to 3 mm, with a pixel and voxel size of less than 1 mm. This will enable us to carry out multiplanar reconstructions.

3.5.3. Breast MRI sequences

3.5.3.1 Morphological sequences

In the past, non-injected T2- and T1-weighted sequences in breast MRI were not considered very useful because of their poor diagnostic value. Since then, many authors have demonstrated the value of using morphological sequences.

T2-weighted sequences can be used to detect cystic lesions, the presence of which indicates benign enhancement, whether annular enhancement in inflammatory cysts or non-mass enhancement in fibrocystic mastopathy (figs. 6 and 7).

T2-weighted sequences with fat saturation are very useful in the case of nipple discharge, making it possible to create indirect MRI galactography images and also improve the detection of small cancers (fig. 8).

T1-weighted sequences without fat saturation are useful for detecting the presence of a fatty component in a lesion, which is an important factor in favour of benignity (fig. 9). These sequences are also useful for confirming the correct position of metal markers in the biopsy site [59] (fig. 10).

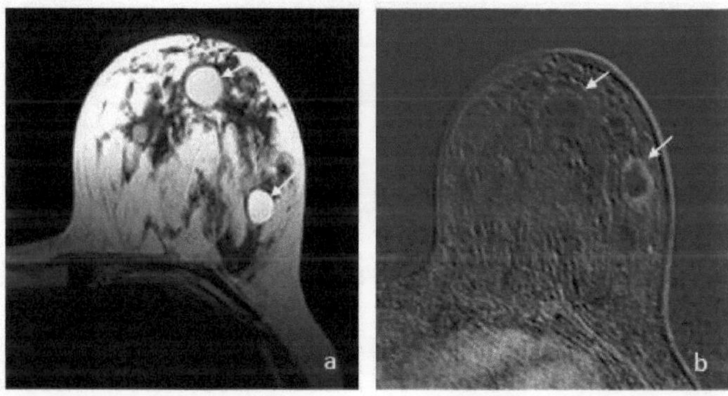

Fig. 6 Inflammatory cysts. (a) T2 sequence, (b) injected subtraction sequence. Round lesions with T2 hypersignal and ring enhancement after injection of contrast medium (arrows).

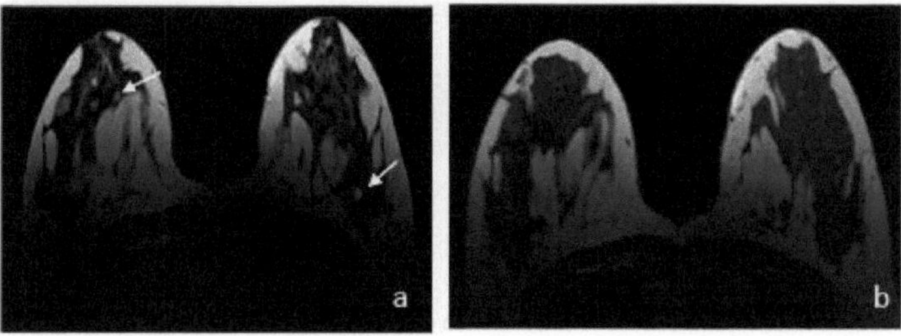

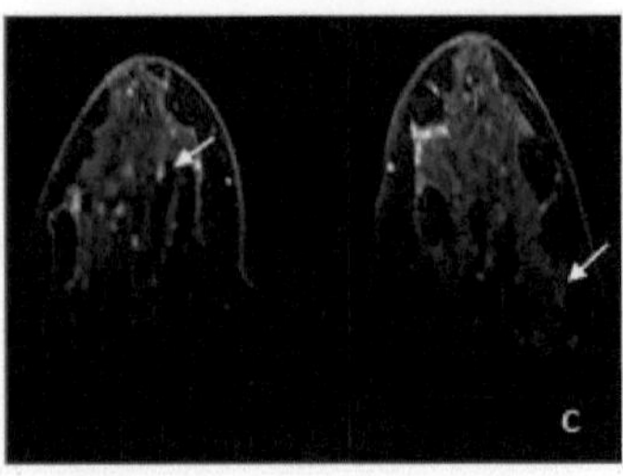

Fig. 7: Fibrocystic mastopathy (a)
T2 sequence, (b) T1 sequence, (c)
T1 Fat Sat sequence after injection of contrast medium. Multiple microcysts in T2 hypersignal, T1 hyposignal with multiple non-mass enhancement after injection of contrast medium (arrows).

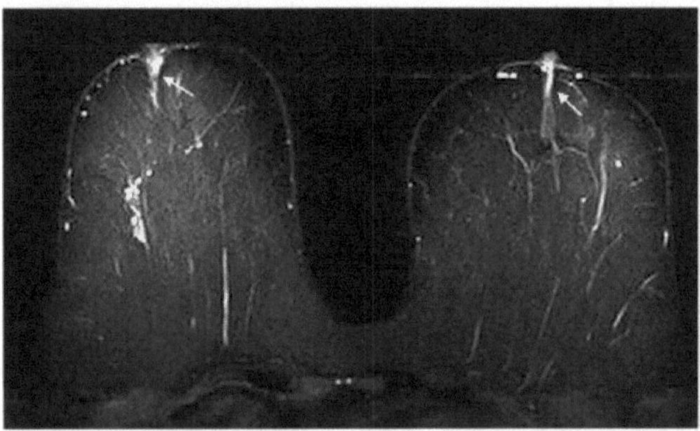

Fig. 8. ductal ectasia. Intracanal hypersignal on T2 sequences with fat suppression (arrows).

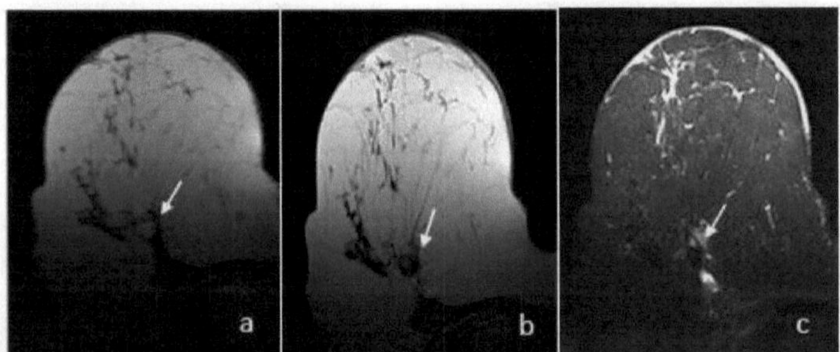

Fig. 9 Cytosteatonecrosis: (a) T1 sequence, (b) T2 sequence, (c) T2 Fat Sat sequence. The lesion is T1 hypersignal, T2 hypersignal and hyposignal on the T2 sequence with fat supression (arrows).

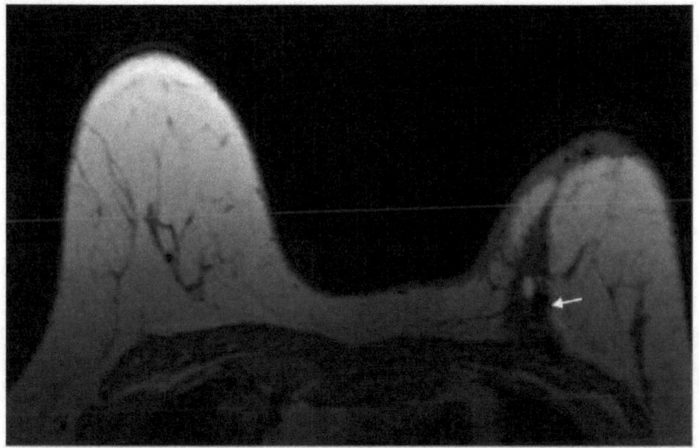

Fig. 10: Position of the metal marker in the T1 sequence (arrow).

3.5.3.2 Dynamic sequences

Dynamic analysis makes it possible to distinguish suspicious abnormal angiogenesis from the various enhancement kinetics. T1 gradient echo sequences after injection of gadolinium chelate (fig. 11).

2D or 3D acquisition?

Compared with 2D sequences, 3D sequences give finer slices with a better signal-to-noise ratio [11]. However, as 3D acquisition is performed without fat suppression, it is advisable to use 2D sequences to reduce the phase encoding artefacts that extend in all three directions in 3D sequences, masking the contours and making it difficult to detect these artefacts on subtraction sequences.

The 3D sequence enables the lesion to be analysed in volume (measurement in the 3 planes, distance from the nipple-areolar plate and the deep plane pectoral) (fig.12).

3.5.3.3 Complementary sequences

o Distribution

The principle of diffusion imaging is to quantify the movement of water molecules in tissues. The objectives of diffusion sequences are to optimise the detection of small lesions and improve the characterisation of benign and malignant lesions. Diffusion MRI can also be used to assess the response to neoadjuvant chemotherapy. An increase of more than 10% in ADC coefficients at the end of the first cycle of chemotherapy indicates a decrease in cell density, and is therefore predictive of response to treatment [60, 61].

o Magnetic resonance spectroscopy

Spectroscopy is a molecular imaging technique. Its principle is to detect an abnormal choline peak in malignant tumours (resonance at 3.2 ppm) [62]. Bartella et al. reported that the addition of spectroscopy to the standard protocol improved the PPV of biopsies from 35% to 82% ($p<0.01$) and enabled biopsy to be avoided in 57% of lesions [63]. In addition, a number of studies have shown that this sequence can demonstrate an early response (at 24 h) to neoadjuvant chemotherapy [64].

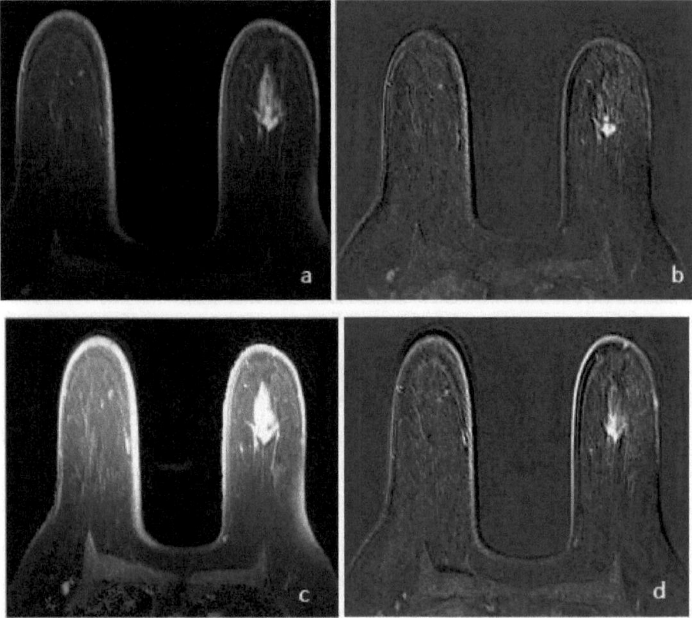

Fig. 11. Enhancement analysis of a malignant tumour in the left breast.
Dynamic analysis enabled the tumour to be distinguished from the rest of the fibroglandular parenchyma by acquisition before the second minute in three-dimensional (3D) T1 weighting (a) and 3D T1 injection with subtraction (b). At six minutes, it is difficult to differentiate the cancer from the breast parenchyma on the injected 3D T1 (c) and injected 3D T1 with subtraction (d) sequences.

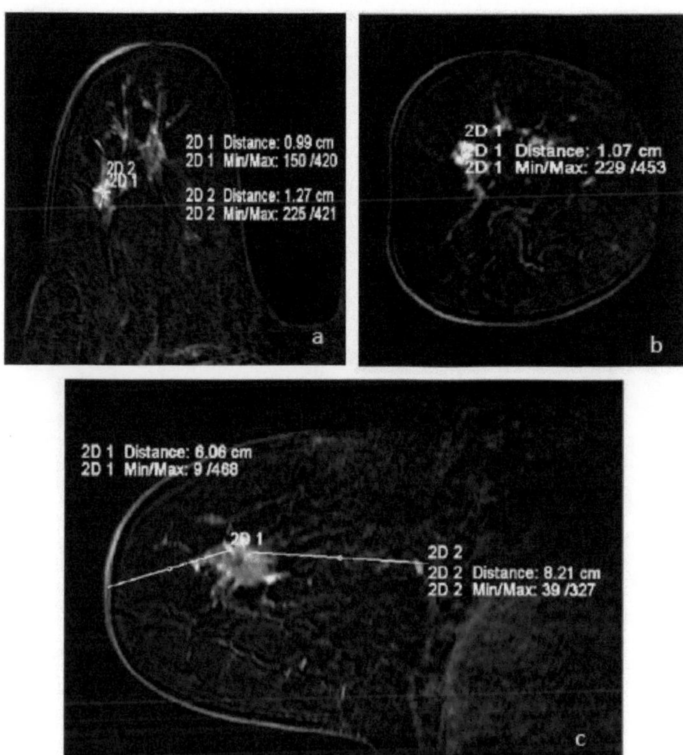

Fig. 12. Injected 3D T1-weighted sequence with subtraction. Analysis the volume of the lesion (measured in the 3 planes (a + b), the distance of the lesion from the nipple-areolar plate and the deep pectoral plane (c).

3.5.4. Specific protocols according to clinical indications

3.5.4.1. Breast implants

As a rule, the image acquisition protocol should include T1- and T2-weighted sequences with selective silicone suppression, which are often useful for distinguishing silicone leaks from periprosthetic fluid effusion [page 374]. A Turbo Spin Echo T2 (TSE T2) sequence with selective suppression of water is used to search for intracapsular rupture, and an STIR sequence with suppression of the fat and water signal is used to detect silicone leaks in the case of extracapsular rupture [page 374] (fig. 13).

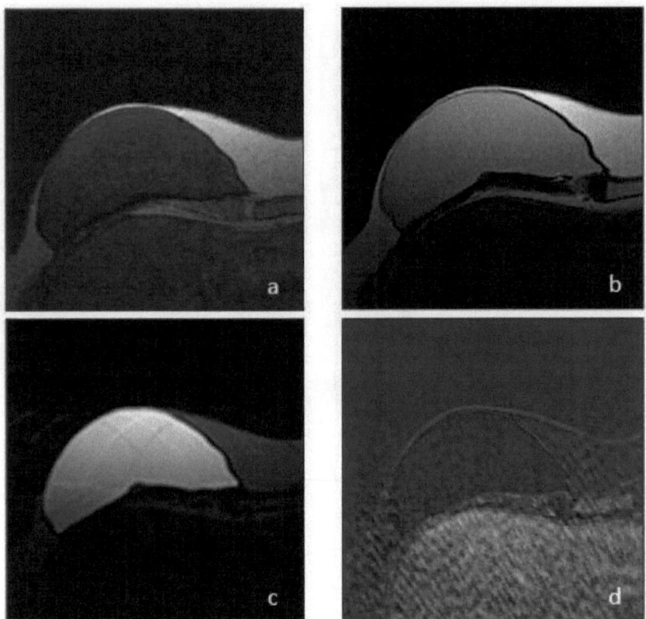

Fig. 13. Appearance of the breast prosthesis in the different sequences. T1-weighted sequence (a), T2-weighted sequence (b), STIR sequence (c) and injected subtraction sequence (d).

3.5.4.2. Breast discharge

A T2-weighted sequence with fat saturation can be used to study the milk ducts. These sequences provide an indirect image of galactography, using the spontaneous contrast of the dilated galactophoric ducts, which appear in T2 hypersignal after fat saturation (fig. 14).

Direct ducto-MRI consists of opacifying the pathological ductus galactophoricus by catheterisation of the pore through which a flow is visualised. Opacification is performed by injecting either physiological saline and analysis is performed on the T2-weighted CISS (constructive interference in steady state) sequence, or gadolinium chelate and analysis is performed on the T1-weighted sequences with fat saturation. However, this technique is rarely used in current practice due to the difficulties of catheterisation, which are similar to those of galactography (10% failure rate).

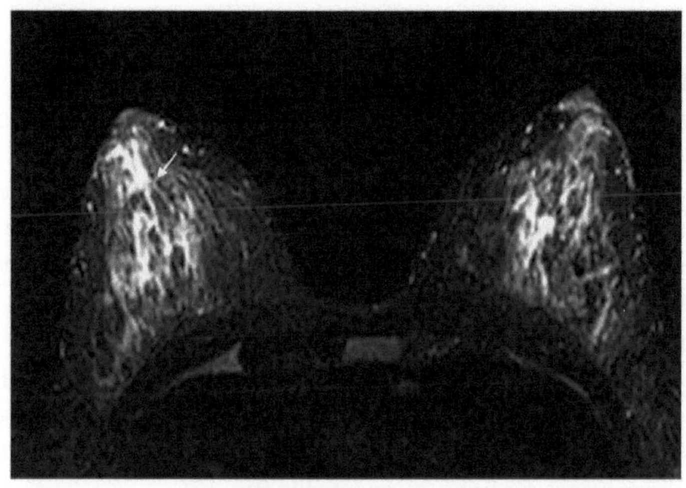

Fig. 14. Breast flow. T2-weighted sequence with fat saturation. Retroareolar intracanal hypersignal (arrow).

4. Anatomy-MRI correlations

The anatomy of the breast can be demonstrated very well with breast MRI. It enables deep areas of the breast to be assessed, such as the deep muscles and the chest wall. Certain structures, such as vessels and lymph nodes, are easily visible, especially after injection of contrast medium. Knowledge of the normal anatomy of the breast on MRI is fundamental to the correct interpretation of the examination.

4.1. Nipple

Contrast enhancement of the nipple is present in 50% of cases [3] and should not be considered pathological in the absence of suggestive clinical signs. These enhancements sometimes extend to the retro-nipple region and the bilateral nature of these images confirms their normality (fig. 15).

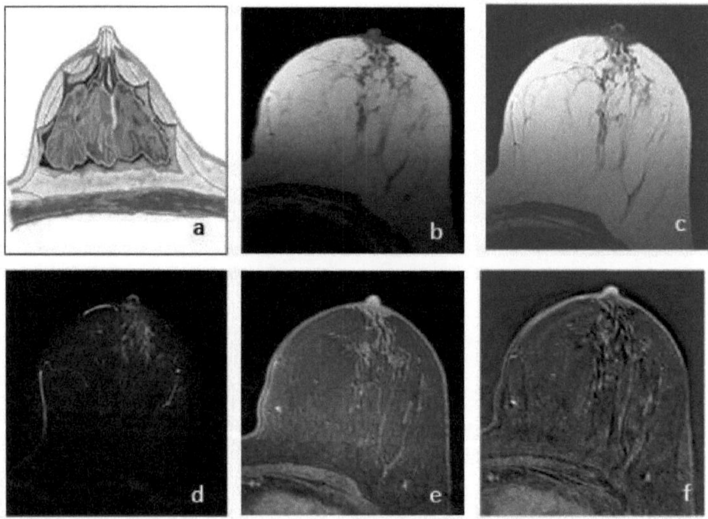

Fig. 15. Nipple. Diagram (arrow) (a), T1-weighted sequence (b), T2-weighted sequence (c), T2 Fat Sat sequence (d), T1 Fat Sat injected sequence (e) and subtracted injected sequence (f).

4.2. Galactophore ducts

Galactophore ducts are not spontaneously visible, except in the case of galactophore ectasia, which are visualised as retroareolar ductal structures converging towards the nipple, the signal from which varies according to their content (fig. 16).

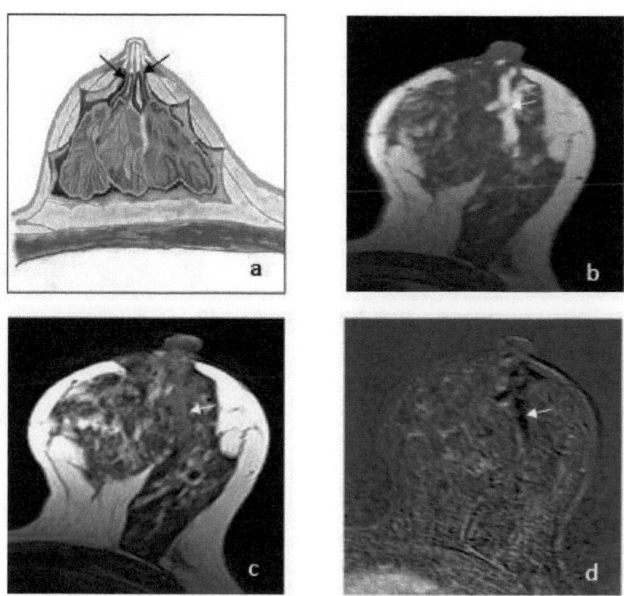

Fig. 16 Galactophoric dilatation. Diagram (arrows) (a), sequence in T1-weighted sequence (b), T2-weighted sequence (c) and injected subtraction sequence (d). Ductal ectasia with protein content in T1 hypersignal, T2 hyposignal, not enhanced after injection of contrast medium (arrows).

4.3. Adipose tissue

The adipose tissue appears hypersignal on T1 and T2 weighted sequences, TSE T2 hyposignal with fat suppression and unenhanced after intravenous injection of contrast medium (fig. 17). The subcutaneous fat is partitioned by the suspensory ligaments of the breast known as Cooper's ligaments in the extension of Duret's fibro-glandular ridges.

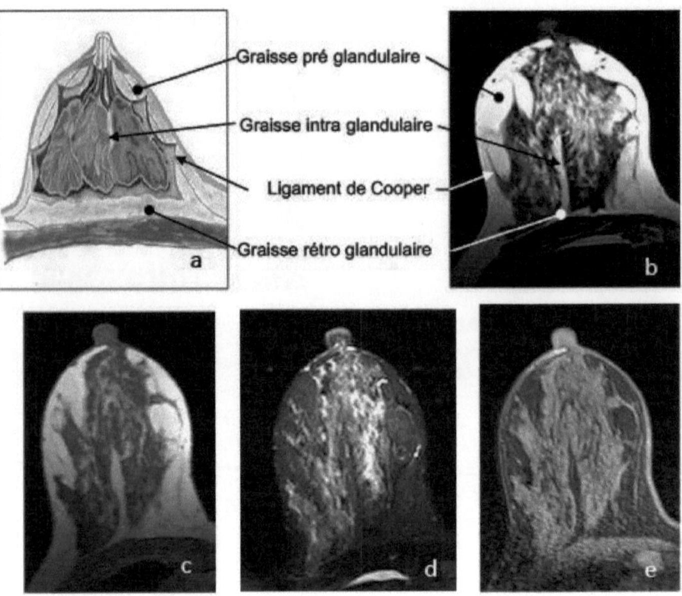

Cooper's ligament
Pre-glandular fat Intra-glandular fat
Retroglandular fat

Fig. 17. adipose tissue. Diagram (a), T2-weighted sequence (b), T1-weighted sequence (c), T2 Fat Sat sequence (d) and T1 Fat Sat injected sequence (e). Adipose tissue in T2 and T1 hypersignal, not enhanced after injection of contrast medium.

4.4. Fibro-glandular tissue

Fibro-glandular tissue is a normal component of the breast. It can be assessed on T1 and T2 weighted sequences and must be quantified according to the BIRADS lexicon in four categories [65]: A. Fatty breast; B. Scattered fibro-glandular tissue; C. Heterogeneous fibro-glandular tissue; D. Dense fibro-glandular tissue (fig. 18).

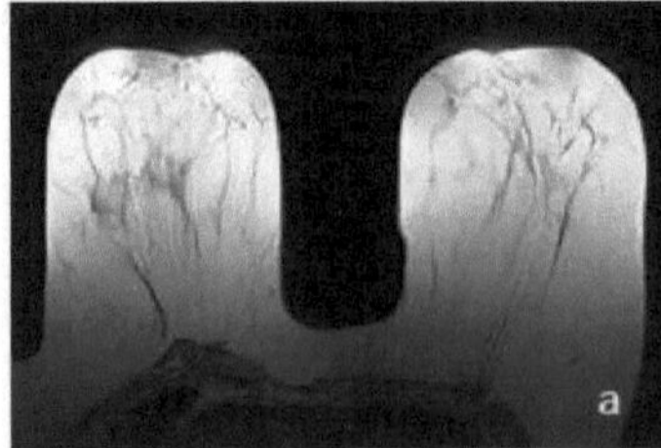

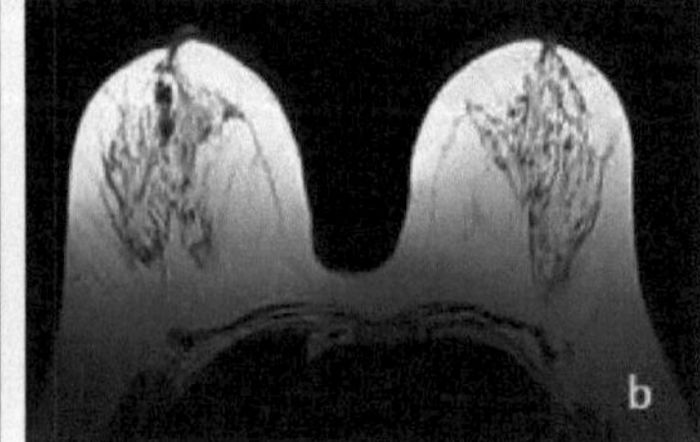

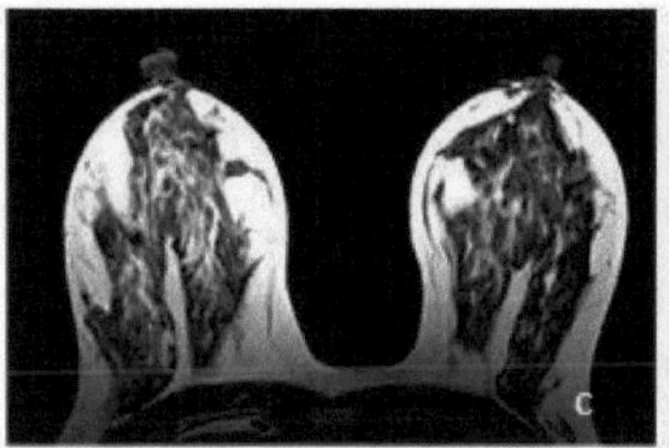

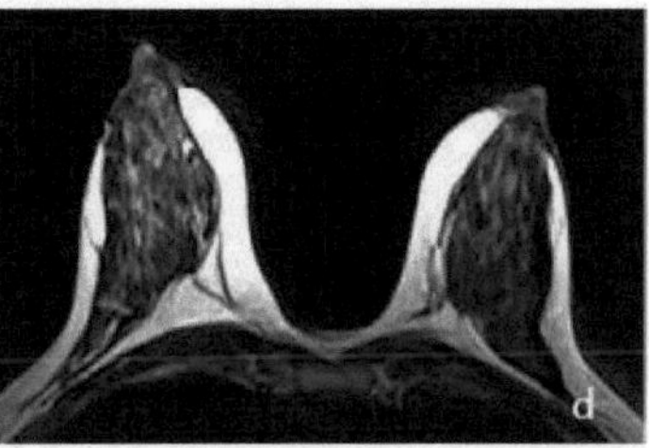

Fig. 18. Breast density according to the ACR BI-RADS classification. T2-weighted sequences: (a) fatty breast, type A; (b) sparse fibro-glandular tissue, type B; (c) heterogeneous fibro-glandular tissue, type C; (d) dense fibro-glandular tissue, type C: Heterogeneous fibro-glandular tissue, type C; (d): Dense fibro-glandular tissue, type D.

On T1 sequences with fat suppression and after injection of gadolinium chelate, the fibro-glandular tissue may be enhanced. This physiological enhancement can be described according to the BIRADS lexicon in four levels: A. minimal; B. slight; C. moderate, and D. marked (fig. 19). Matrix enhancement is assessed 90 seconds after injection, at the time when malignant lesions are enhanced, to determine whether this matrix enhancement may be masking cancer. In general, matrix enhancement is progressive and may spread throughout the breast. However, it is plausible to observe very early, rapid and intense fibroglandular enhancement. Whatever the phase of the cycle, matrix enhancement is possible and may persist after the menopause. Matrix enhancement is not directly related to the amount of glandular tissue. A patient with dense breasts may show little or no matrix enhancement. On the other hand, a patient with sparse fibro-glandular tissue may have marked matrix enhancement. The level of matrix enhancement must be reported in the report.

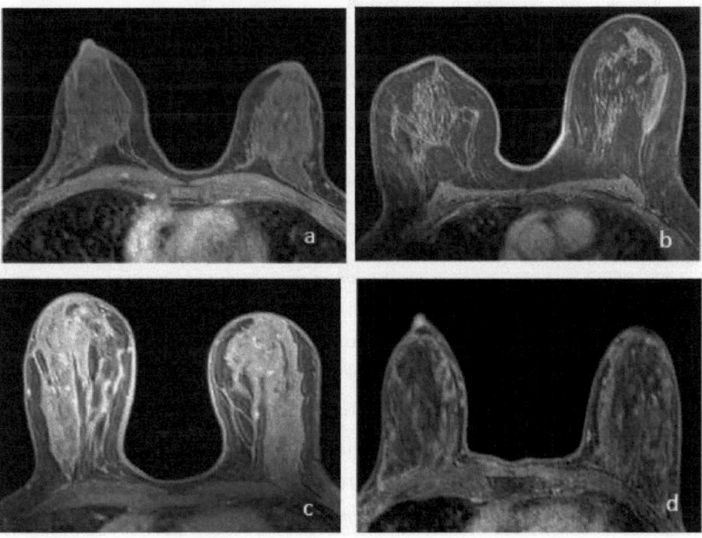

Fig. 19. Physiological enhancement of fibroglandular breast tissue. T1 sequences injected with fat suppression in four levels according to the BIRADS lexicon: minimal (a), slight (b), moderate (c) and marked (d).

4.5. Muscles

The muscles show an intermediate signal on morphological T1 and T2 sequences. The muscles are poorly enhanced after injection of contrast medium. Axial and sagittal sections clearly show the posterior adipomuscular interface, revealing its integrity or its involvement by posterior cancers (fig. 20).

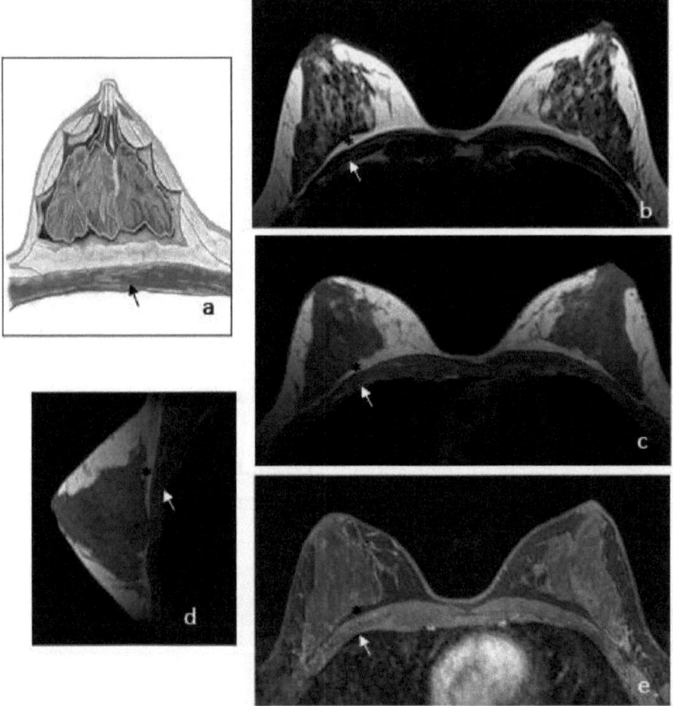

Fig. 20. Pectoralis muscle. Diagram (a), T2-weighted sequence (b), T1-weighted sequence, axial section (c), sagittal section (d) and native T1 injected sequence (e). The pectoralis muscle is in intermediate T2 and T1 signal, slightly enhanced after injection of contrast medium (arrow). Posterior adipomuscular interface (asterisk).

4.6. Vessels

The breast receives its blood flow from several sources. The lateral thoracic artery comes from the axillary artery and supplies the upper external quadrant of the breast, accounting for around 30% of the vascularisation of the breast (fig. 21). Sixty per cent of the vascularisation of the breast comes from the internal mammary artery and its perforating branches, which supply the central and internal part of the breast (fig. 21). The remainder of the vascular supply comes

mainly from the branches of the intercostal arteries. The vessels are easily identified, and may be visible along part of their course in the slice, or follow their course in several successive slices. Maximum intensity projection (MIP) images can also help to confirm the trajectory of the vessels (fig. 22).
The spontaneous signal of the vessels, particularly in T2, and their enhancement are variable. These variations are linked to the speed of the flow within the vessel and its orientation in relation to the slice plane.

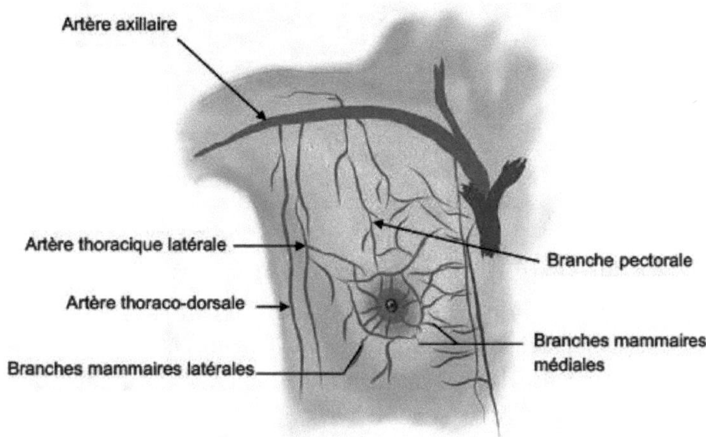

Axillary artery
Lateral thoracic artery
Thoracodorsal artery
Medial mammary branches
Pectoral branch
Lateral mammary branches

Fig. 21. Vascularisation of the breast.

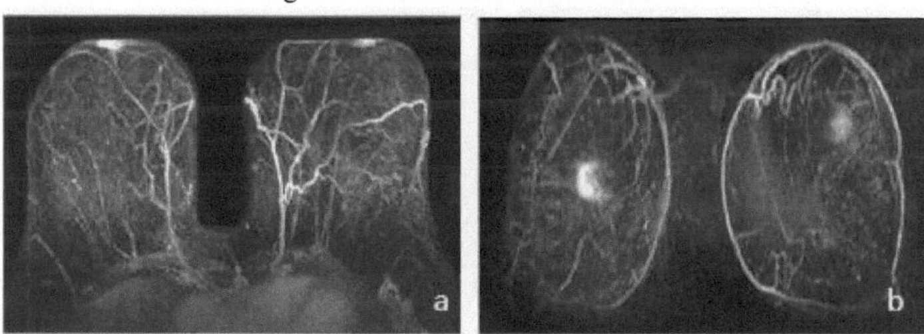

Fig. 22. Maximum intensity projection (MIP) reconstruction. (a) axial section, (b) coronal section

4.7. Lymph nodes

Lymphatic drainage of the breast is mainly from lateral and medial trunks extending from the areola to the armpit (97%), with the internal mammary chain accounting for the remaining 3% [66]. Berg's level I lymph nodes are located below the pectoralis minor muscle. Level II lymph nodes are located behind the pectoralis minor muscle, and level III lymph nodes are located above the pectoralis minor muscle (fig. 23).

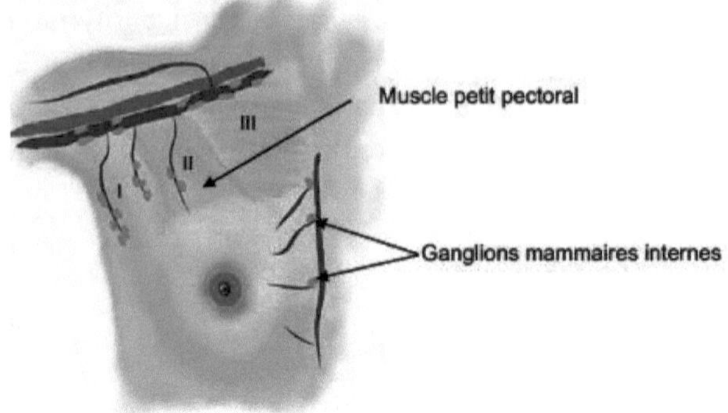

Small pectoral muscle
Internal mammary nodes
Fig. 23. The three Berg lymph node levels and the internal mammary nodes.

Nodes are encountered in most MRI scans. Their topography is usually behind or in the external extension of the pectoralis major muscle. Intramammary lymph nodes are easily diagnosed with their kidney-shaped appearance, with sharp, regular contours, in T1 and T2 hypersignal, and their fatty hilum in T1 and T2 hypersignal. Contrast enhancement is usually early, rapid and moderate (fig. 24). However, lymph nodes can present a diagnostic dilemma [67] when morphological criteria are not typical. The dynamic curve may be unreliable, often mimicking malignant lesions. T2-weighted images with fat suppression may be useful in these cases, as the signal intensity of the lymph nodes is greater than that of normal glandular parenchyma.

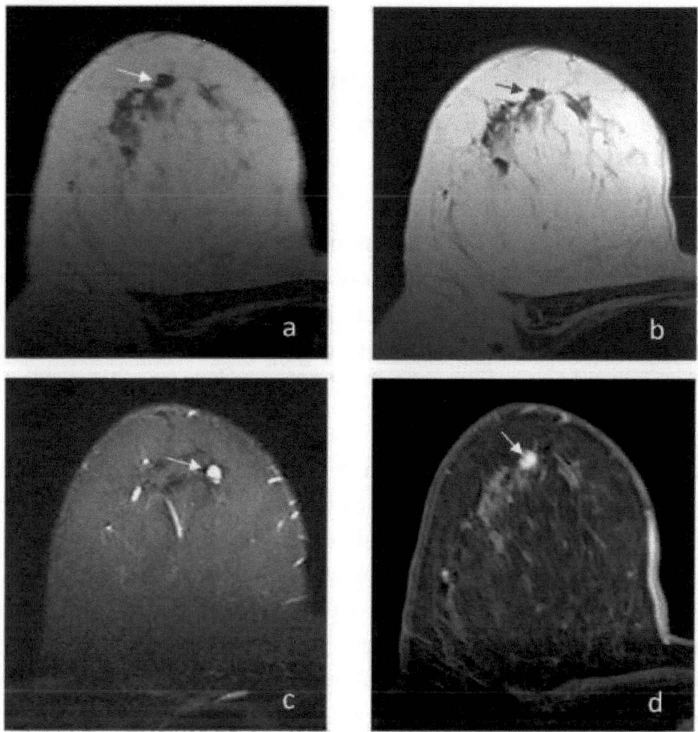

Fig. 24. Intramammary ganglion. T1-weighted sequence (a), T2-weighted sequence (b), T2 Fat Sat sequence (c) and T1 injected sequence (d). Reniform intramammary ganglion, with clear and regular contours, in T1 and T2 hyposignal, T2 Fat Sat hyper signal and enhanced after injection of contrast medium with a fatty hilum in T1 and T2 hypersignal (arrows).

5. Principles of breast MRI interpretation

It is based on the ACR BI-RADS lexicon [65]. It comprises a morphological analysis and a dynamic analysis.

5.1. Morphological analysis

Morphological analysis is carried out on the first series subtracted so that glandular enhancement does not interfere with interpretation, without forgetting to look at the native sequences which are of high resolution and which will give the best view of the contours, internal architecture and internal enhancement. Always compare with non-injected T1 and T2 images.

5.1.1. Focus

This enhancement measures less than 5 mm and does not show up on non-injected sequences (fig. 25). Because of its small size, this enhancement does not allow detailed morphological analysis or dynamic analysis. It is usually secondary to a benign pathology such as focal fibrocystic mastopathy, intramammary ganglion or adenofibroma. The risk of malignancy of these lesions is low, around 3% [68]. Elements in favour of the benign nature of foci are their symmetrical nature, associated with T2 microcysts, and the absence of associated mammographic or ultrasound signs (fig. 26). Their degree of suspicion increases in the case of a neighbouring malignant lesion or in the context of exploration of a high-risk breast (fig. 27).

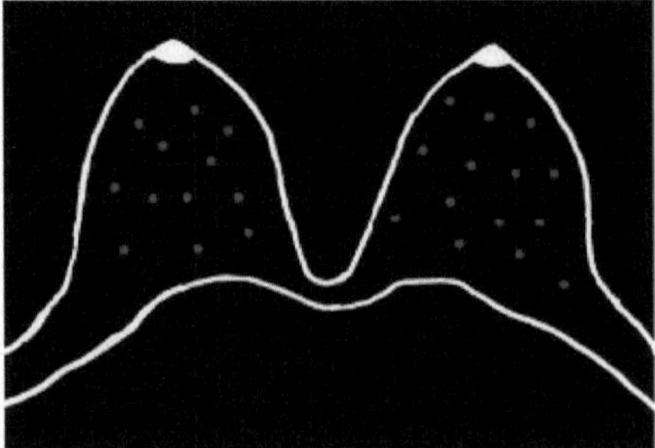

Fig. 25. Diagram of foci

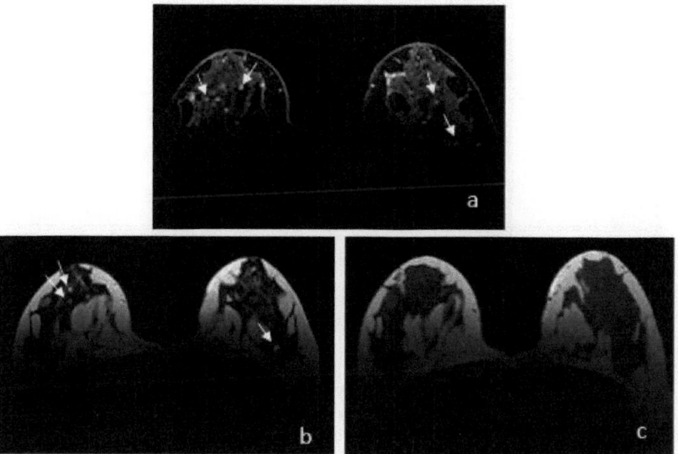

Fig. 26. Multiple foci secondary to fibrocystic mastopathy. Injected subtraction sequence (a), T2-weighted sequence (b) and T1-weighted sequence (c). Foci after injection of contrast medium (arrows), presence of T2 hypersignals (microcyst) (arrows).

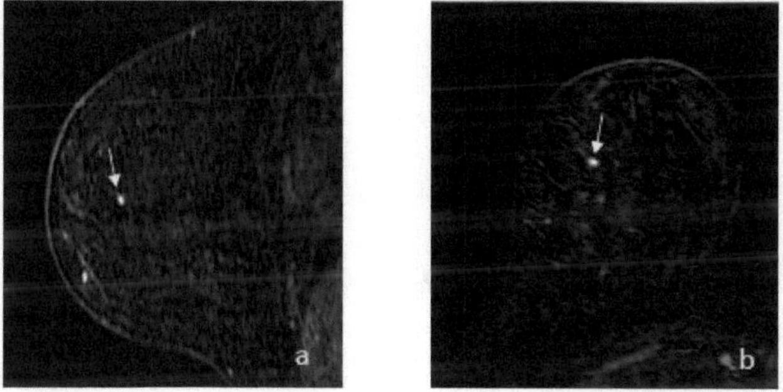

Fig. 27. Single focus in postmenopausal women. T1 injected sequence with subtraction, sagittal section (a), axial section (b).

5.1.2. Mass

A mass is a lesion more than 5 mm in diameter that occupies a volume, usually found on non-injected sequences (fig. 28) [69].

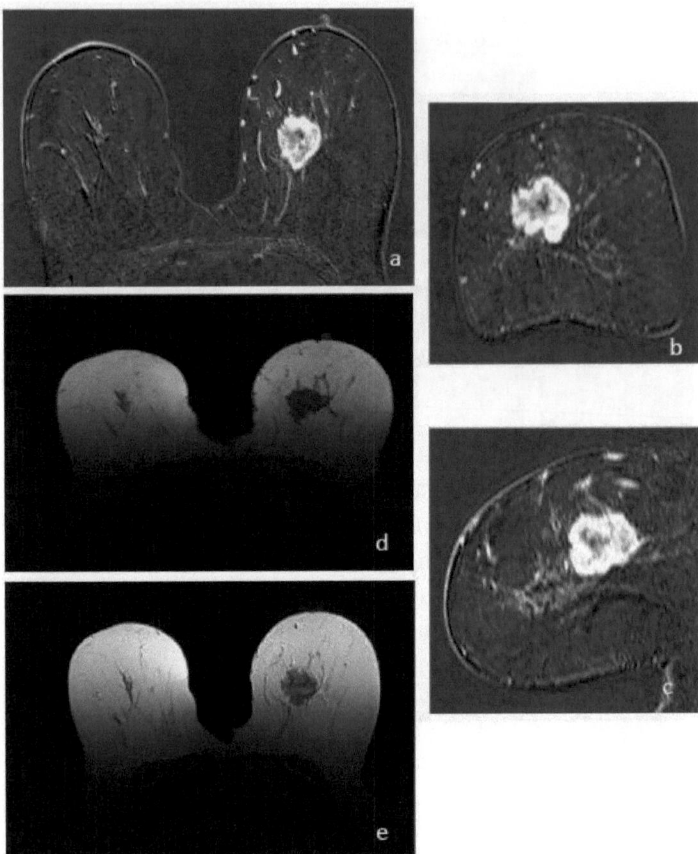

Fig. 28. Mass. T1 injected sequence with subtraction of axial section (a), coronal section (b), sagittal section (c), T1-weighted sequence (d) and T2-weighted sequence (e).

A mass is a volume-occupying enhancement visible on non-injected T1 and T2 sequences.

5.1.2.1.Form

- Oval shape

The oval or elliptical shape favours benignity (fig.29), most often a cyst, fibroadenoma or papilloma (fig. 30). Malignant lesions can present oval shapes such as myxoid carcinomas and also small carcinomas in situ with poorly defined contours.

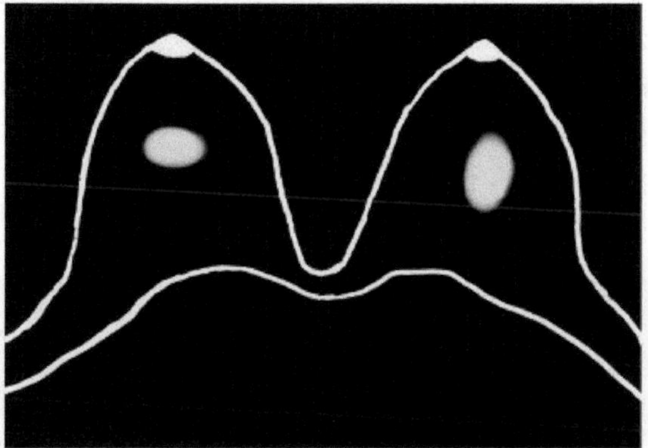

Fig. 29. Diagram, oval-shaped mass.

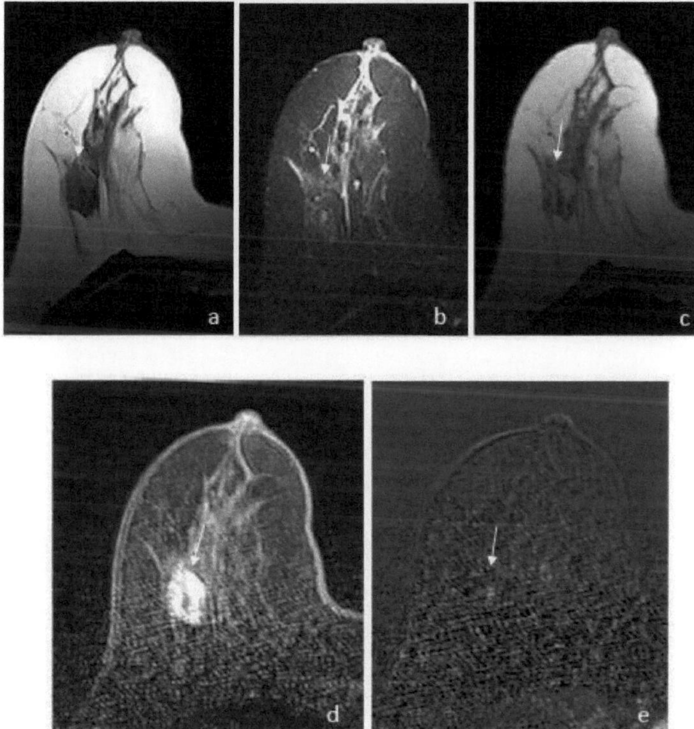

Fig. 30. Oval-shaped mass. T2-weighted sequence (a), T2 Fat Sat-weighted sequence (b), T1 sequence (c), native T1 injected sequence (d) and subtracted injected sequence (e). Shaped mass with T2 hypersignal, T2 Fat Sat hyposignal, heterogeneous T1 hypersignal, homogeneous enhancement on native injected T1 sequences, weakly enhanced on subtracted injected sequences. Internal septa in T1 and T2 hyposignal, not enhanced after injection (arrows). Histology: myxoid fibroadenoma.

- Round shape

The round or spherical shape is defined after injection of contrast medium (fig. 31). As with the oval shape, the round mass is often a cyst, fibroadenoma or papilloma (fig. 32). Less commonly, myxoid or medullary carcinomas may present with a round shape, associated with signs of infiltration of the surrounding tissue.

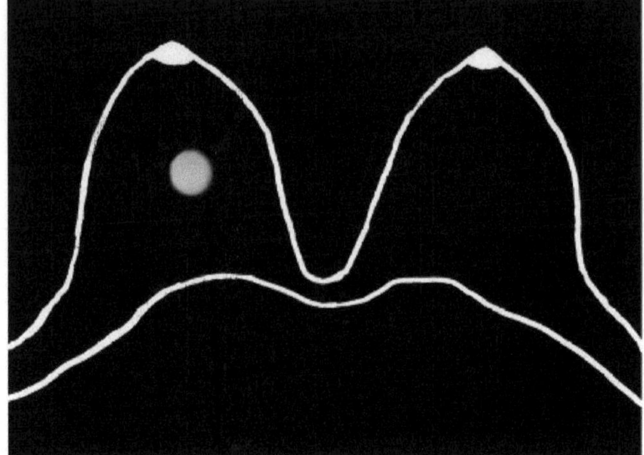

Fig. 31. Diagram, round mass.

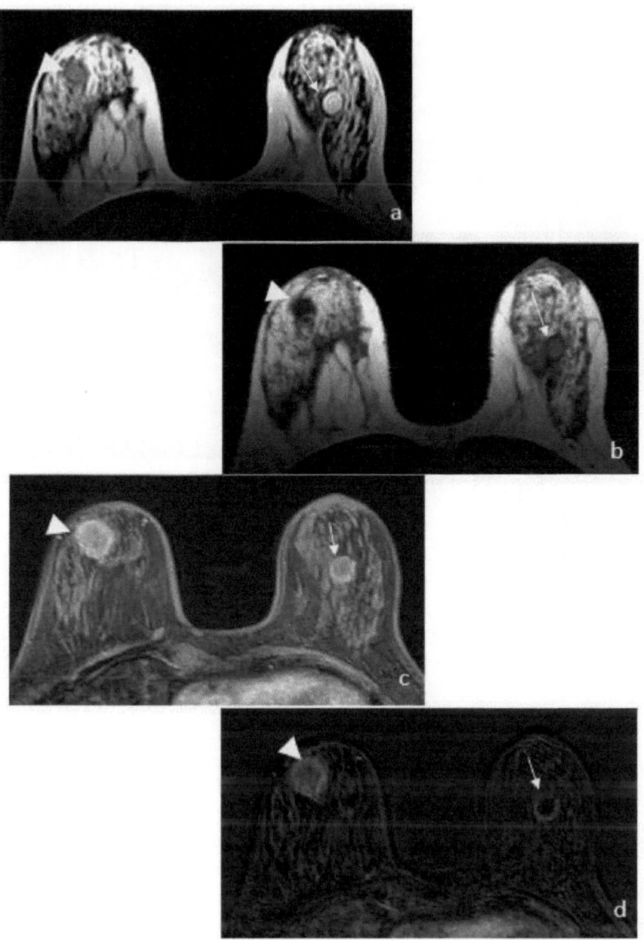

Fig. 32. Round mass. T2-weighted sequence (a), T1-weighted sequence (b), native injected T1 sequence (c) and subtracted injected sequence (d). Two round masses, one in the right breast in T1 and T2 hypopositivity, with heterogeneous enhancement on native injected T1 sequences and subtracted injected sequences.
Histology: non-specific carcinoma (arrowheads). The other in the left breast, hypersignal T2, hyposignal T1, with a thin enhanced wall (arrows). Histology: inflammatory cyst.

- Irregular shape

The shape is neither oval nor round (fig. 33).

Irregularly shaped masses are suggestive of malignancy, usually infiltrating carcinomas (fig. 34). In some cases, benign masses may also have an irregular shape, such as lesions of idiopathic granulomatous mastitis.

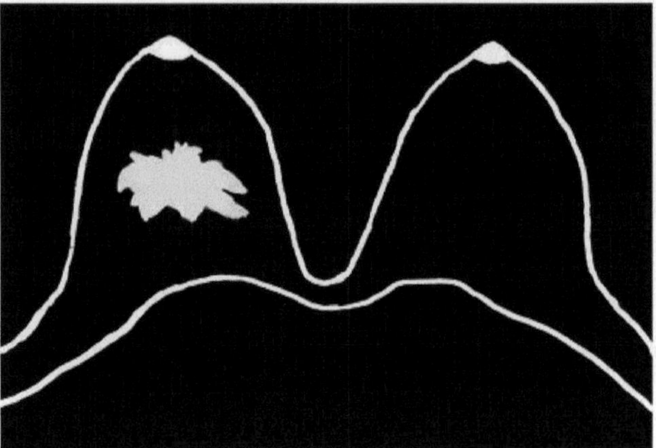

Fig. 33. Diagram, irregularly shaped mass.

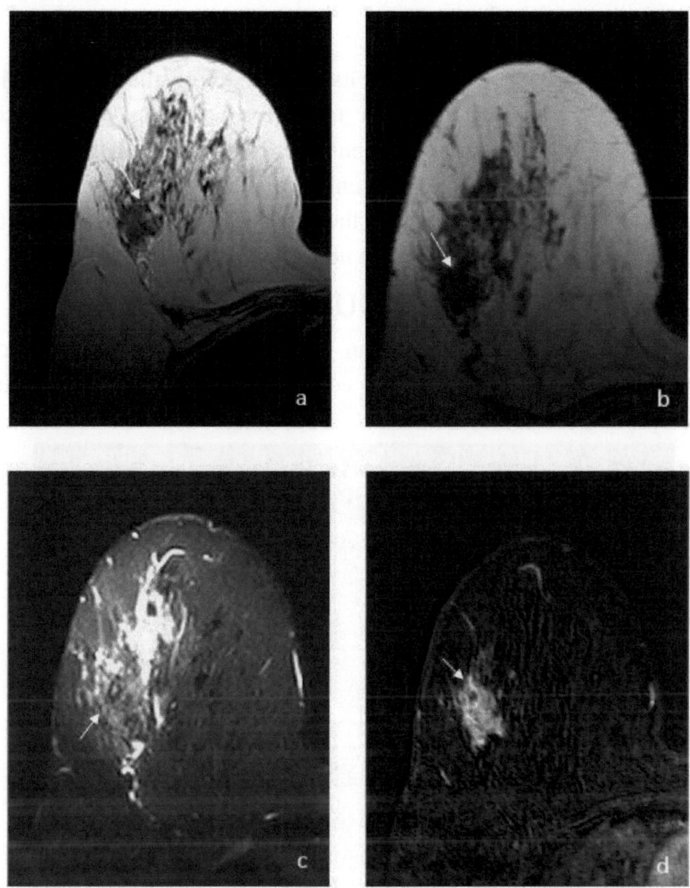

Fig. 34. Irregularly shaped mass. T2-weighted sequence (a), T1-weighted sequence (b), T2 Fat Sat sequence (c) and injected subtraction sequence (d). Irregular T1- and T2-hyposignal mass with heterogeneous enhancement on injected subtraction sequences (arrows). Histology: non-specific carcinoma.

5.1.2.2 Contours

The contours of a mass correspond to its interface with the adjacent glandular parenchyma. It is therefore essential to perform the analysis on the first subtraction so that glandular enhancement does not interfere with interpretation. In the case of masking glandular enhancement, this interface is poorly individualised. Also, in dense breasts, the mass may be difficult to distinguish from adjacent glandular parenchyma on non-injected sequences.

- Circumscribed contours

Circumscribed masses are benign in 97-100% [70] (figs. 35 and 36). Carcinomas rarely have circumscribed contours and can be seen in mucinous, tubular or medullary carcinomas.

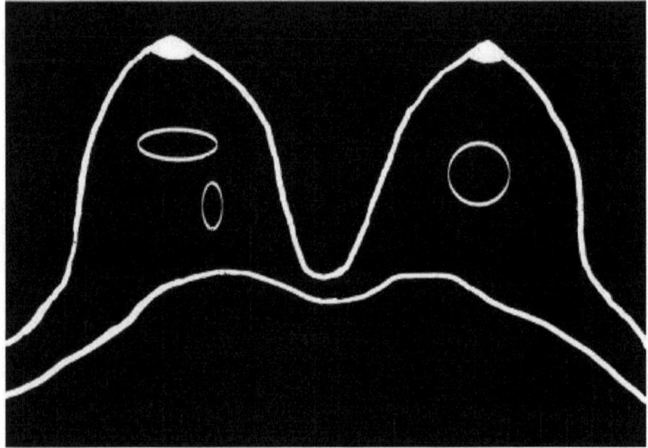

Fig. 35. Diagram, masses with circumscribed contours.

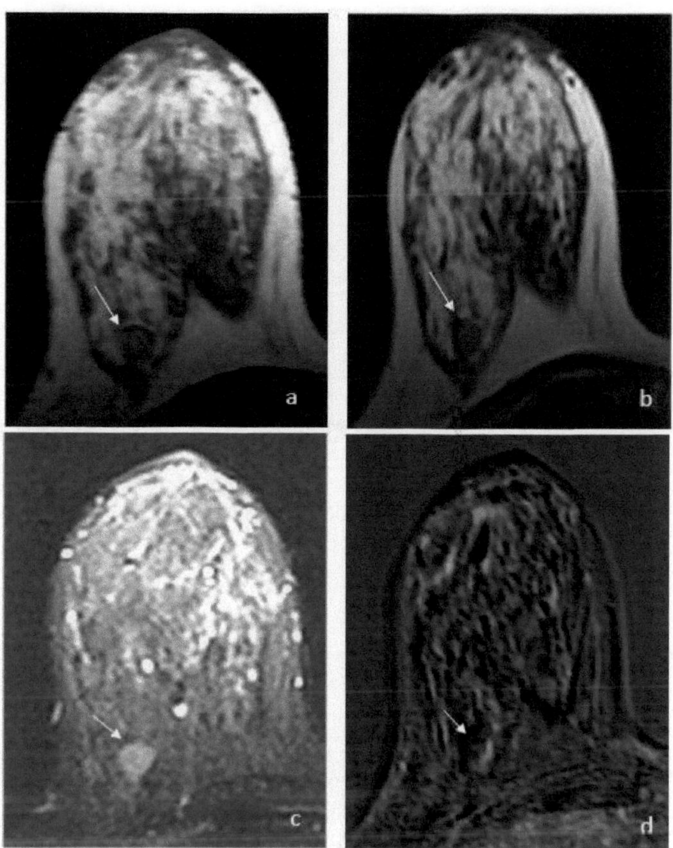

Fig. 36. Mass with circumscribed contours. T2-weighted sequence (a), T1-weighted sequence (b), T2 Fat Sat sequence (c) and injected subtraction sequence (d). Round mass with circumscribed contours, T1 and T2 hyposignal, T2 Fat Sat hypersignal, not enhanced on injected subtraction sequences (arrows). Histology: fibroadenoma.

- Irregular contours

Irregular contours are characterised by thin seepage lines (fig. 37).
Irregular contours are typical of infiltrative carcinomas (fig. 38). Inflammatory masses also tend to have irregular contours (mastitis, abscesses), particularly after percutaneous biopsy.

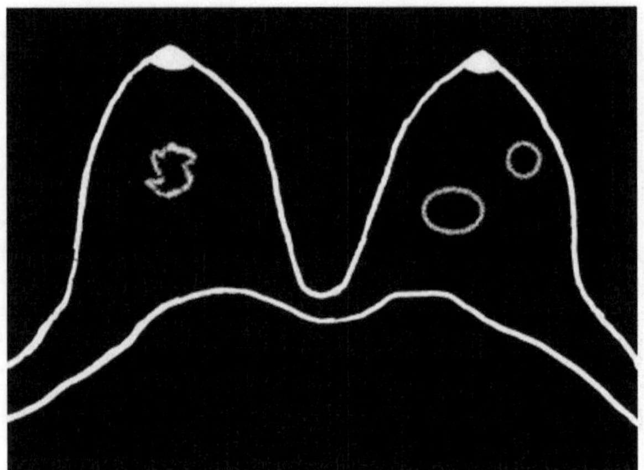

Fig. 37. Diagram, masses with irregular contours.

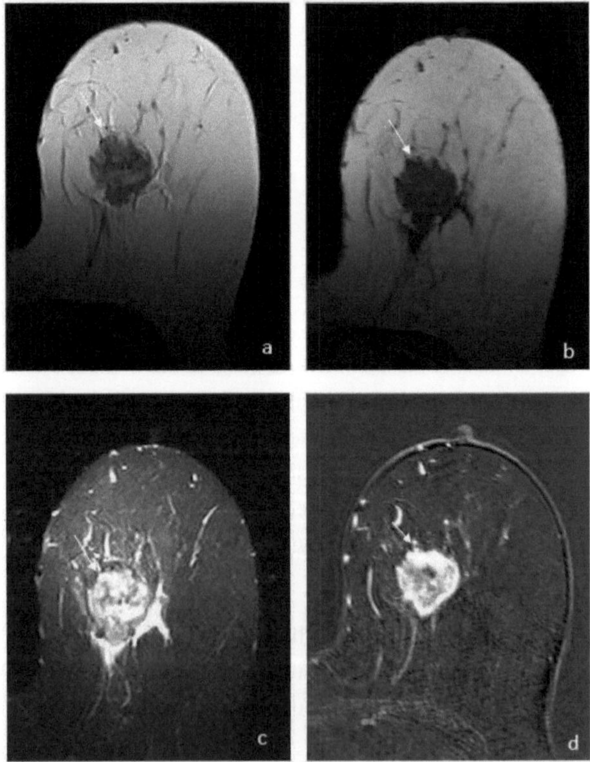

Fig. 38. Mass with irregular contours. T2-weighted sequence (a), T1-weighted sequence (b), T2 Fat Sat sequence (c) and injected subtraction sequence (d). Irregular mass, with irregular contours, in T1 and T2 hypersignal, in T2 Fat Sat hypersignal, surrounded by hypersignal oedema, enhanced on subtraction

injected sequences (arrows). Histology: non-specific infiltrating carcinoma.

- Spiculated contours

Radial extensions can be seen around the edge of the mass (Fig. 39). As with irregular contours, spiculated contours are typical of invasive carcinomas (fig. 40). Some benign lesions, such as radial scarring, have spiculated contours.

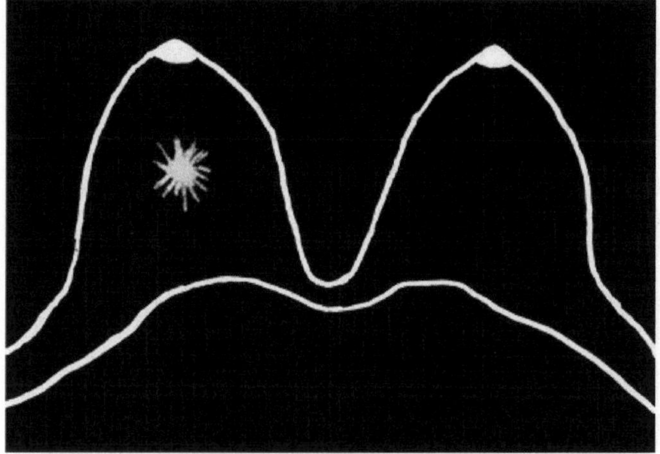

Fig. 39. Diagram, masses with spiculated contours.

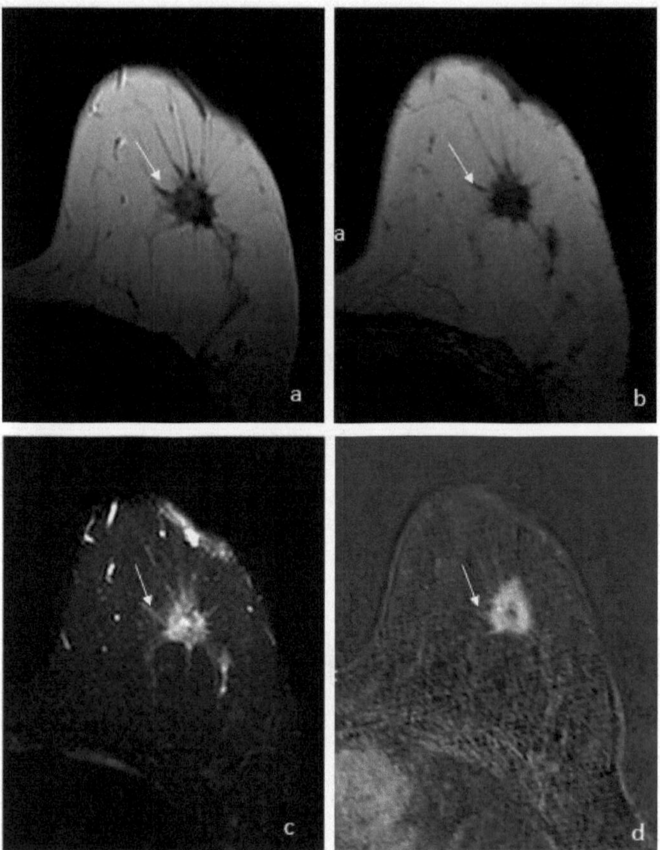

Fig. 40. Mass with spiculated contours. T2-weighted sequence (a), T1-weighted sequence (b), T2 Fat Sat sequence (c) and injected subtraction sequence (d). Irregular mass, with spiculated contours, in T1 and T2 hyposignal, in T2 Fat Sat hypersignal, with heterogeneous enhancement on injected subtraction sequences with the presence of spicules (arrows). Histology: non-specific infiltrating carcinoma.

5.1.2.3 Internal raising

- Homogeneous enhancement

Complete and uniform enhancement of the mass (fig. 41). This type of enhancement is common in benign masses such as fibroadenomas (fig. 42).

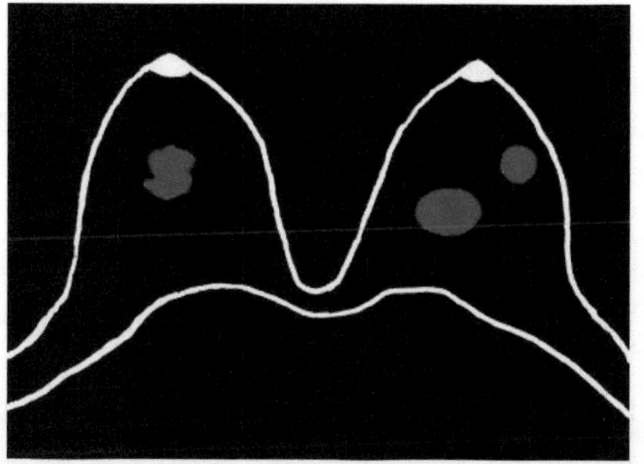

Fig. 41. Diagram, homogeneous enhancement masses.

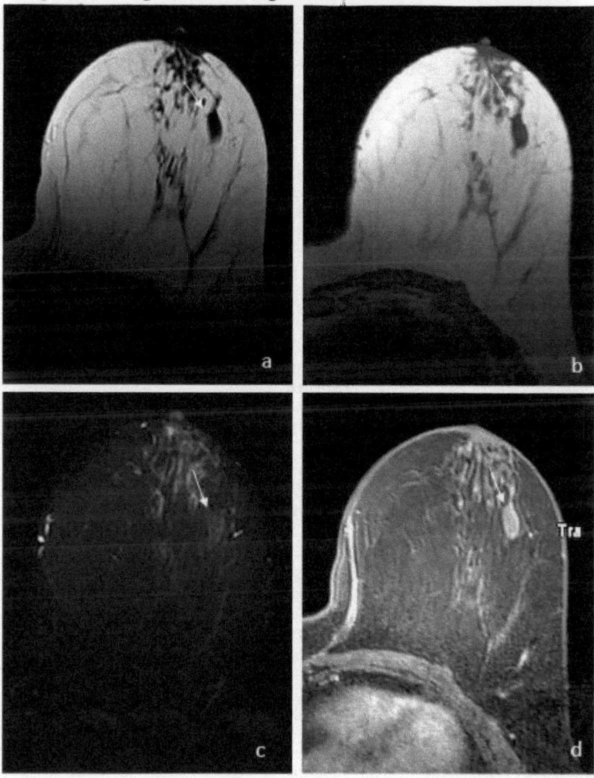

Fig. 42. Homogeneously enhancing mass. T2-weighted sequence (a), T1-weighted sequence (b), T2 Fat Sat sequence (c) and injected T1 sequence (d). Oval mass, with circumscribed contours, in hyposignal T1, T2 and T2 Fat Sat, homogeneously enhanced on injected sequences (arrows). Histology: fibroadenoma.

- Heterogeneous raising

Granular enhancement of the mass (fig. 43). This is a non-specific enhancement and can be found in both benign and malignant lesions (fig. 44). Heterogeneous enhancement is generally less common in malignant lesions, but may be seen in lobular carcinoma.

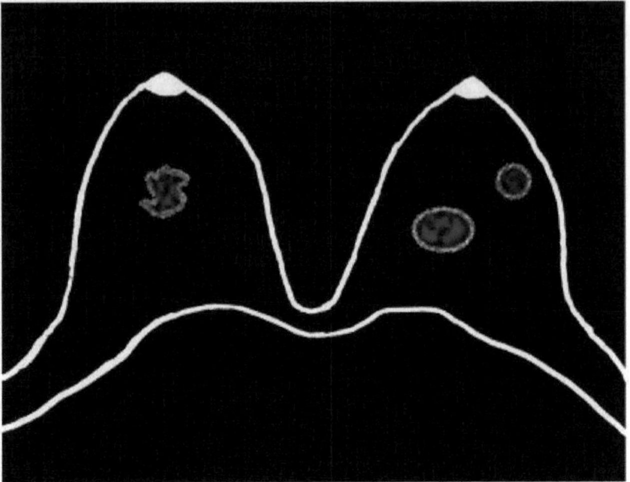

Fig. 43. Diagram, masses of heterogeneous enhancement.

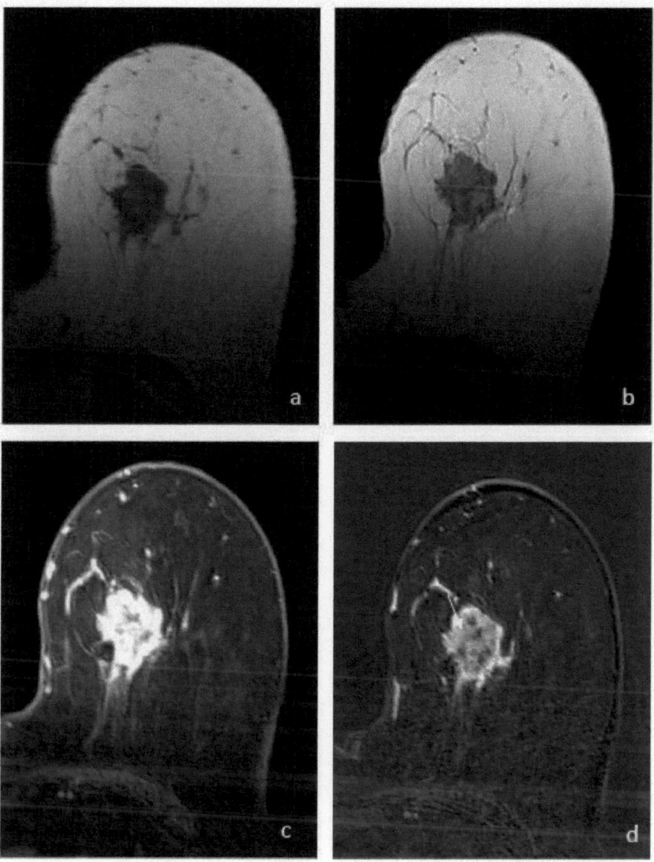

Fig. 44. Mass with heterogeneous enhancement. T2-weighted sequence (a), T1-weighted sequence (b), native injected T1 sequence (c) and subtracted injected sequence (d). Mass of irregular shape and contours, in T1 and T2 hypopositivity, with heterogeneous enhancement on injected sequences (arrow). Histology: non-specific infiltrating carcinoma.

Ring enhancement is a centripetal enhancement, from the periphery towards the centre (fig. 45). This enhancement is highly suggestive of cancer but has a low prevalence in small lesions (20%) [68] (fig. 46).

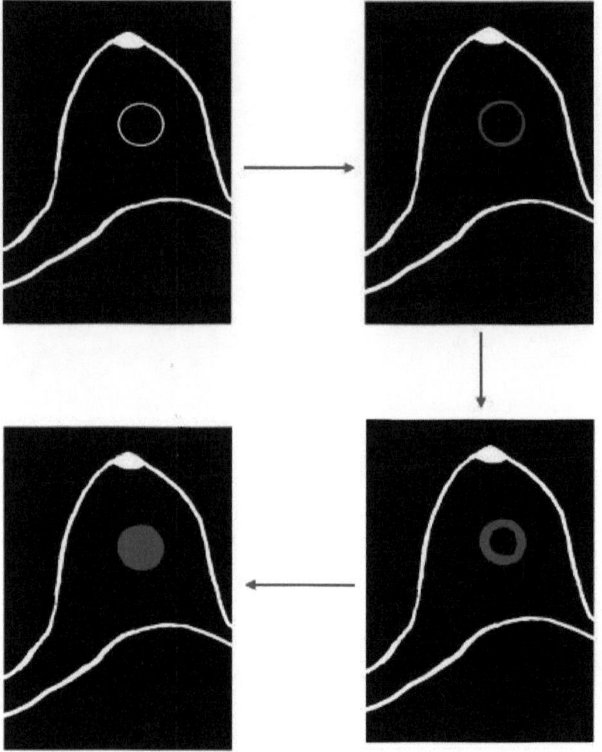

Fig. 45. Diagrams, annular enhancement.

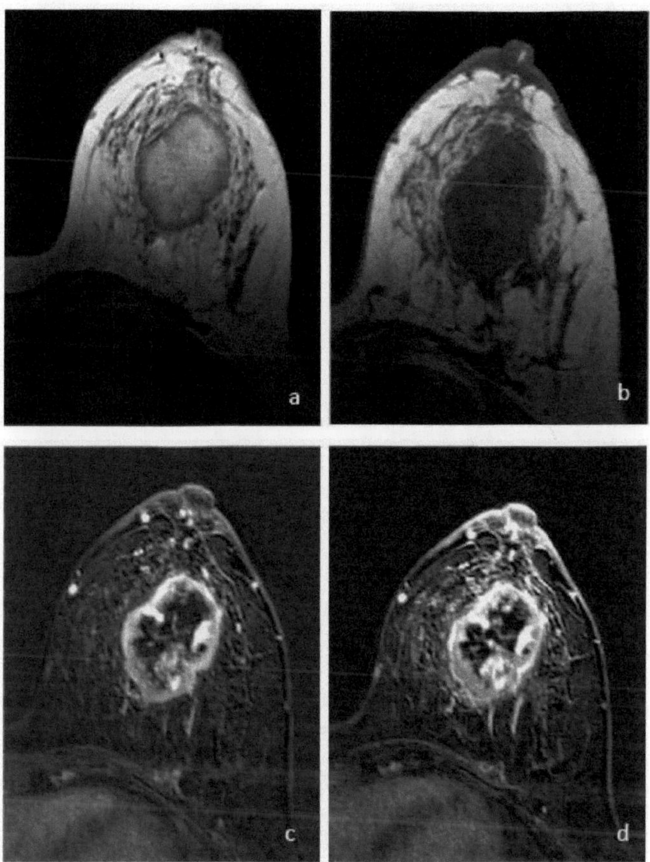

Fig. 46. Annular enhancement mass. T2-weighted sequence (a), T1-weighted sequence (b), native injected T1 sequence (c) and subtracted injected sequence (d). A mass of irregular shape and contours, with T1 hypersignal, T2 hypersignal and annular enhancement on injected sequences (arrows). Histology: non-specific infiltrating carcinoma.

Centrifugal enhancement, from the centre towards the periphery (fig. 47). This type of enhancement is more compatible with benign lesions, especially if it is associated with other benign signs such as circumscribed contours, absence of peri-lesional swelling, etc (fig. 48).

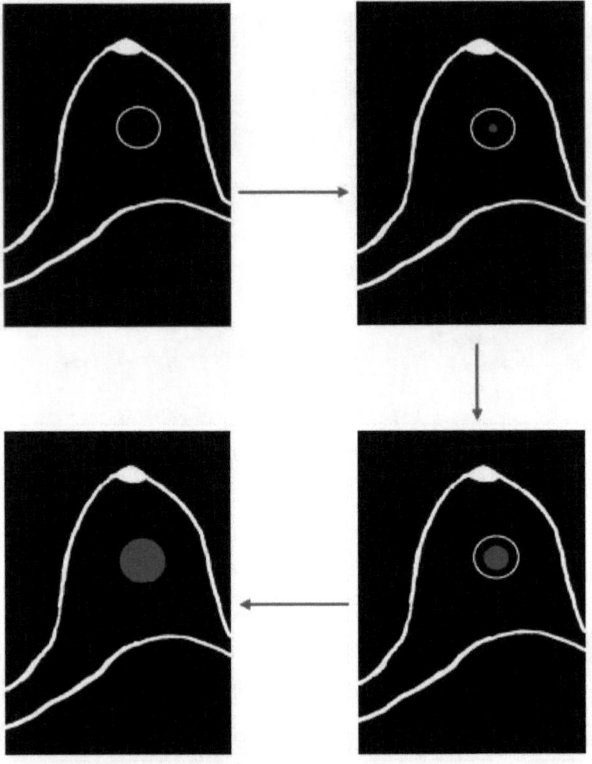

Fig. 47. Diagrams, central elevation.

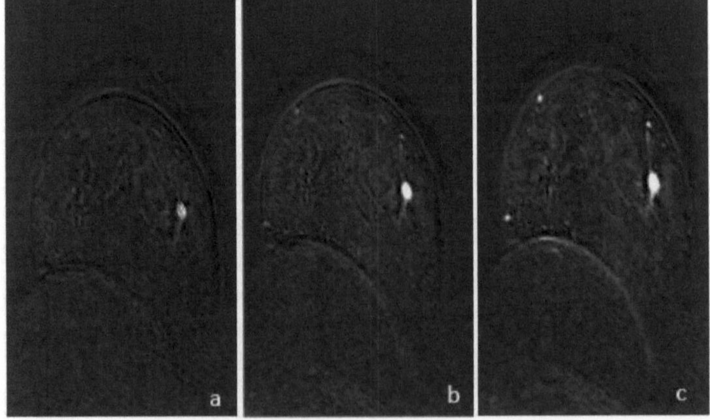

Fig. 48. Central enhancement mass. Subtracted sequences injected (a+b+c). Round mass with circumscribed contours and central enhancement on injected sequences. Histology: fibroadenoma.

Raising the internal septa

Raised internal septa can be seen in inflammatory lesions such as abscesses or in malignant lesions (figs. 49 and 50).

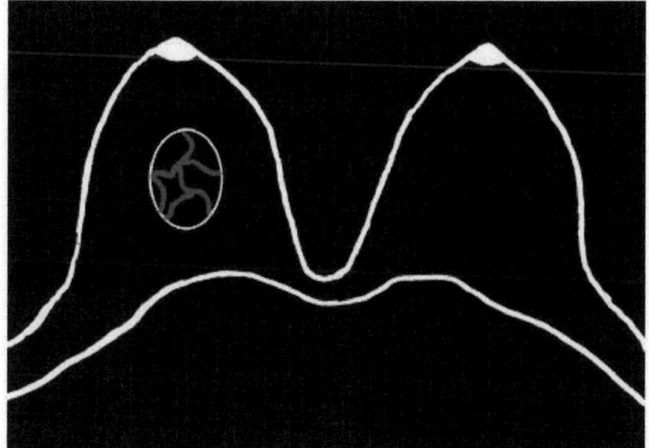

Fig. 49. Diagram, enhancement of the internal septa.

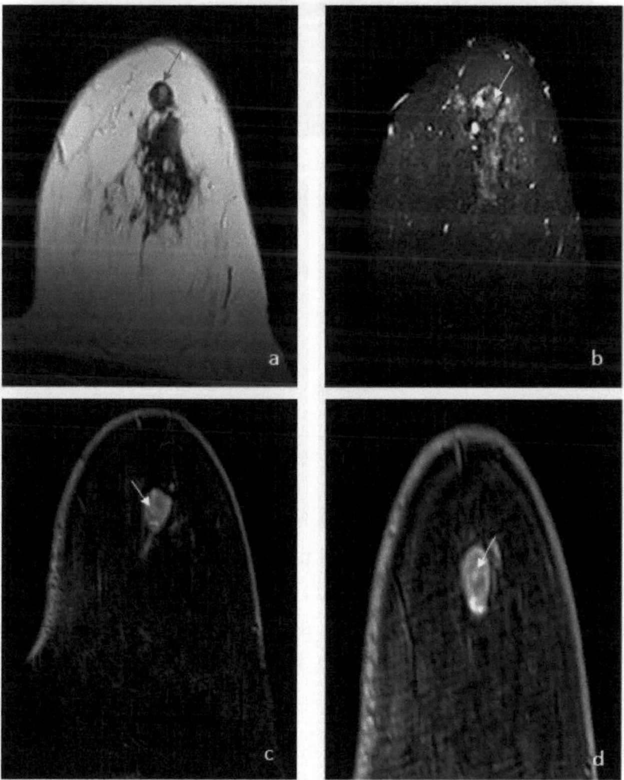

Fig. 50. Lesion with enhanced medial septae. T2-weighted sequence (a), T2 Fat

Sat-weighted sequence (b) and injected subtraction sequence (c+d). Round mass with circumscribed contours, hypersignal T2 and T2 Fat Sat, showing septae in hyposignal T2 and hyposignal T2 Fat Sat, enhanced after injection of contrast medium (arrows). Histology: cyst with septae.

- No enhancement of the internal septa

Non-enlarged internal walls are suggestive of an adenofibroma or fibrocystic mastopathy [68] (figs. 51 and 52). Non-enhanced septations are considered to be benign (> 95%) [70].

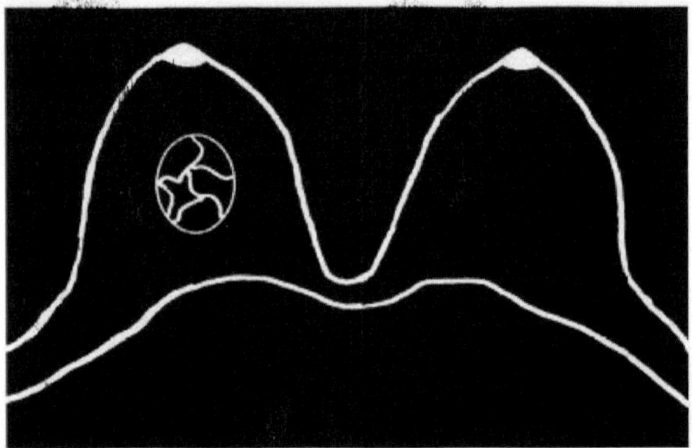

Fig. 51. Diagram of the unenhanced internal septa.

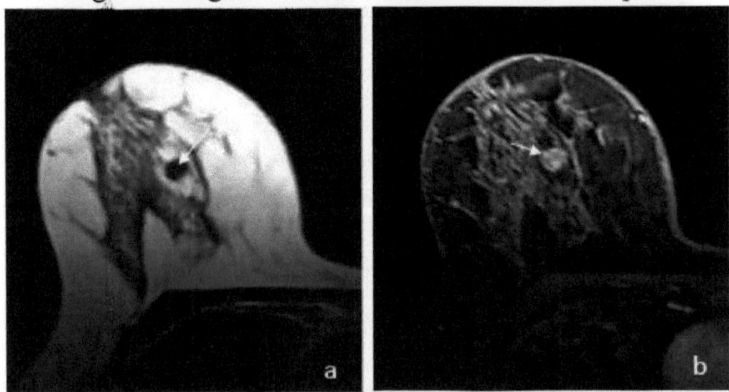

Fig. 52. Lesion with unenhanced medial septa. Weighted sequence T2 (a), T1 injected sequence (b). Round mass with circumscribed contours, low-positivity T2, with low-positivity T2 septa, not enhanced after injection of contrast medium (arrows). Histology: fibroadenoma.

5.1.3. Raising without mass

A non-mass enhancement is an area of enhancement that is neither a mass nor a vessel. This enhancement does not occupy a volume and cannot be seen on non-injected T1 and T2 sequences. This enhancement is detected on post-injection sequences (fig. 53). This enhancement must be confirmed on the native injected images, in order to rule out displacement artefact. Non-mass enhancement may be found in carcinoma in situ, lobular carcinoma, fibrocystic mastopathy secondary to hormonal or inflammatory variations [11, 69, 71].

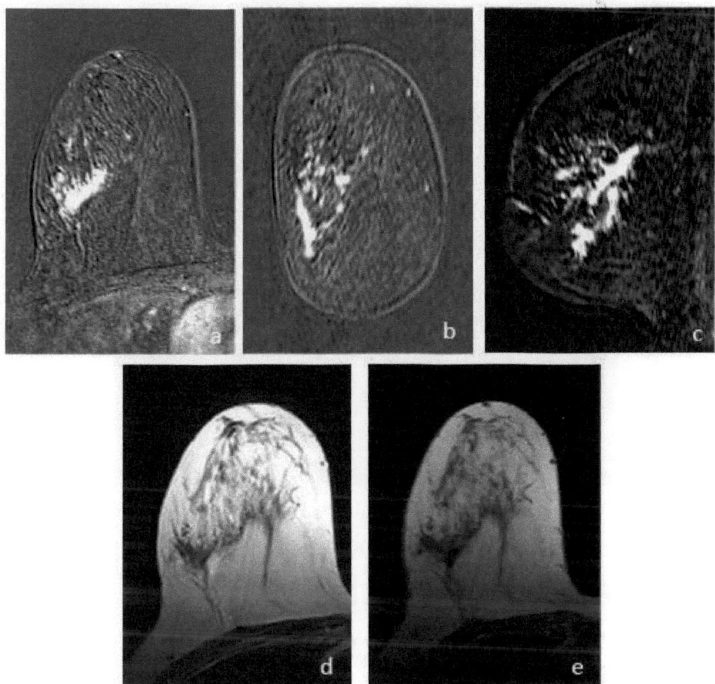

Fig. 53. Non-mass enhancement. Subtracted injected sequences (a+b+c), T2-weighted sequence (d), T1-weighted sequence (e). Non-mass enhancement not occupying a volume in space (arrows), not visible on morphological T1 and T2 sequences. Histology: infiltrating lobular carcinoma.

The description of a non-mass enhancement includes a study of the distribution and internal characteristics of the enhancement, and must be compared with the contralateral breast.

5.1.3.1.Distribution

- Focal" non-mass enhancement

An increase of less than 25% in the volume of a breast quadrant (fig. 54).

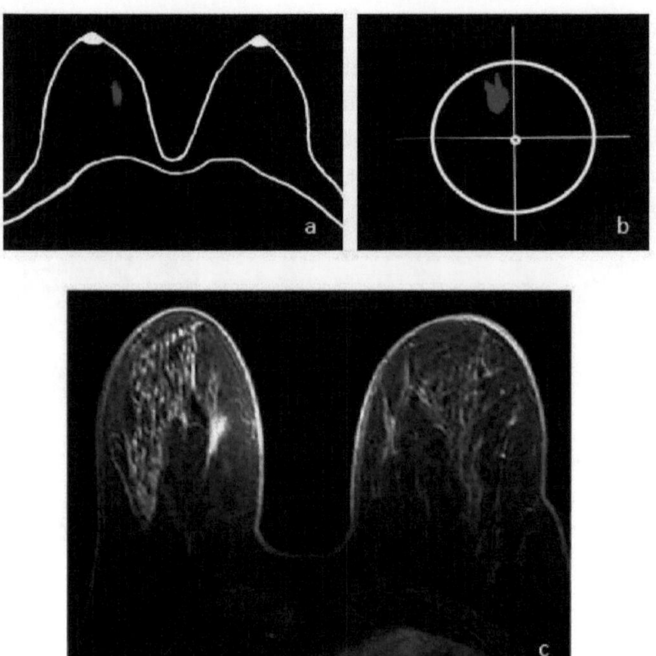

Fig. 54. Focal non-mass enhancement. Diagrams (a+b), injected subtracted sequences (c).

- Linear" non-mass enhancement

The enhancement must be linear in two orthogonal planes and punctiform in the third plane (fig. 55). It may or may not converge towards the nipple. Linear non-mass enhancement is essentially a sign of ductal pathology, either carcinomatous such as non-specific carcinoma in situ, atypical such as atypical hyperplasia, or benign such as ectatic galactophoritis [72] (fig. 56).

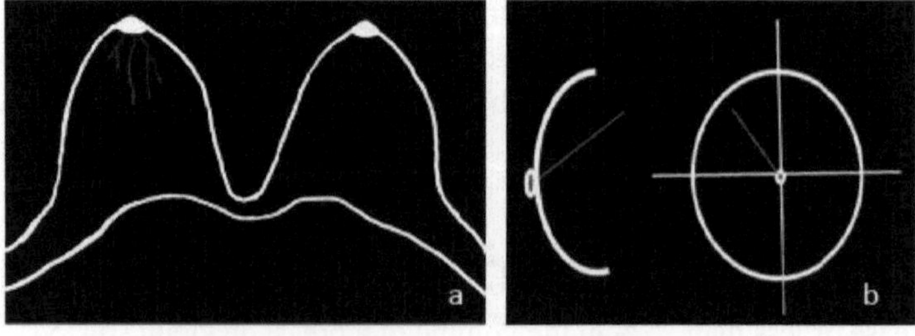

Fig. 55. Diagrams, linear non-mass enhancement (a+b).

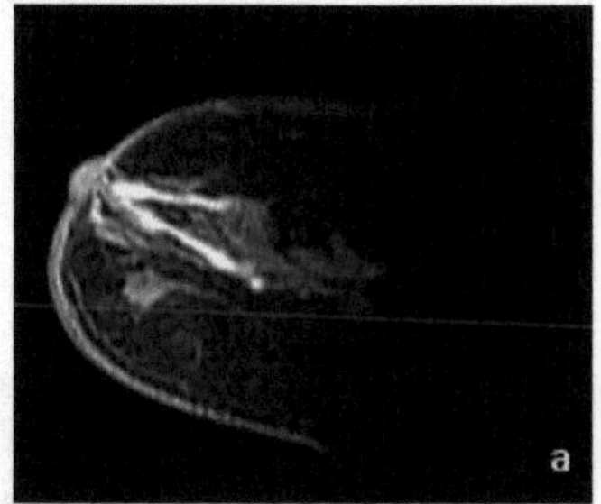
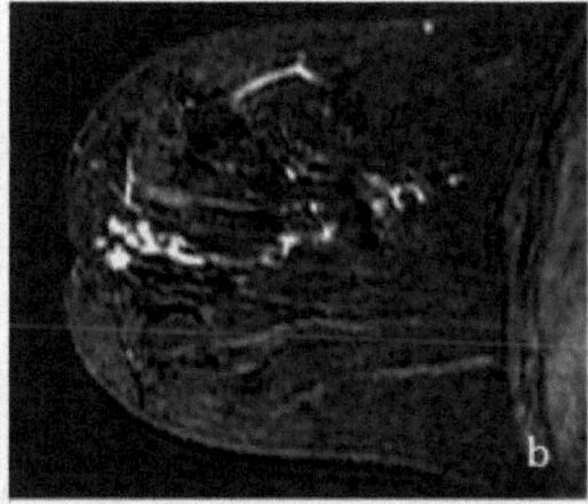

Fig. 56. Linear non-mass enhancement. Subtracted sequences injected sagittal sections (a+b), linear non-mass enhancement, converging towards the nipple.

- Segmental" non-mass enhancement

Triangular or conical enhancement, oriented towards the nipple, showing a galactophoric network (fig. 57). Segmental non-mass enhancement is the most suspicious of the non-mass enhancements. Its PPV is high in most studies in the literature at 67-100% [73]. Non-mass enhancement is most often indicative of malignant disease (fig. 58).

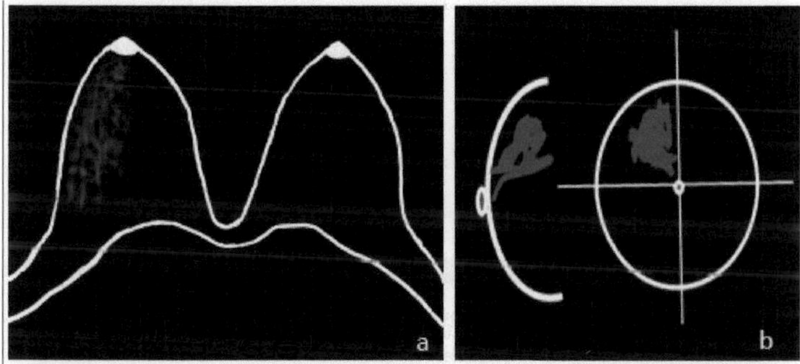

Fig. 57. Diagrams, enhancement without segmental mass (a+b).

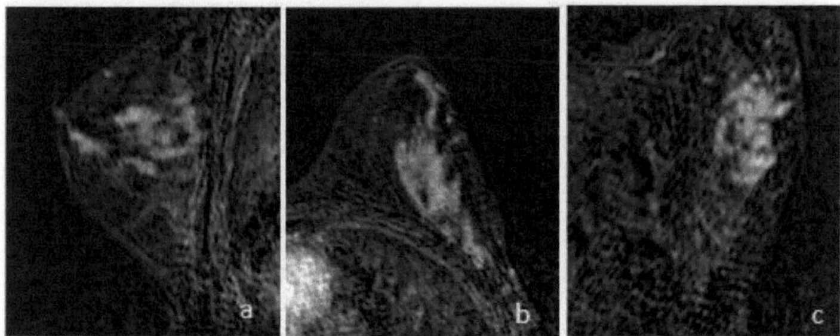

Fig. 58. Segmental non-mass enhancement. Subtracted sequences injected, sagittal section (a), axial section (b) and coronal section (c). Non-massive triangular enhancement, converging towards the nipple.

- Regional" non-mass enhancement

Enhancement of more than 25% of a breast quadrant, possibly single or multiple, with no particular orientation (fig. 59). This type of enhancement is associated with a 21% probability of infiltrating lobular carcinoma, more rarely with non-specific infiltrating carcinoma [70] (fig. 60).

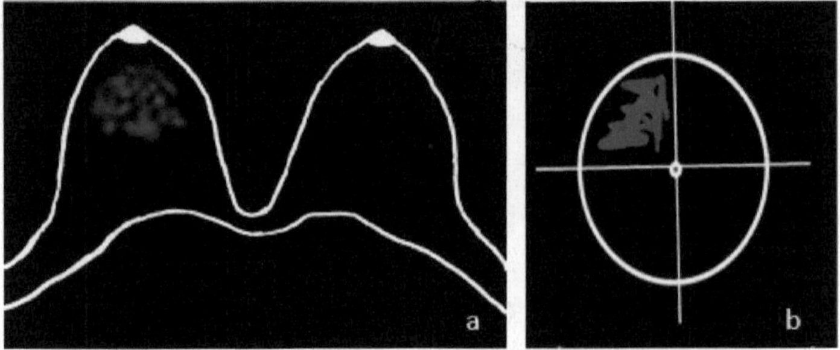

Fig. 59. Diagrams, regional non-mass enhancement (a+b).

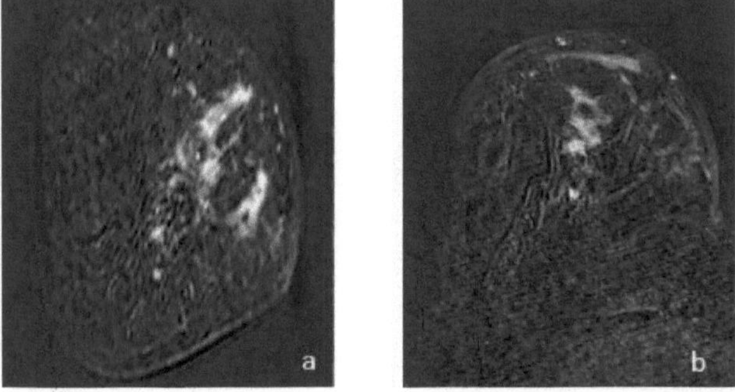

Fig. 60. Regional non-mass enhancement. Subtracted sequences injected, Coronal section (a) and axial section (b). Extensive non-mass enhancement, with no particular orientation.

Unilateral enhancement of uniform and regular distribution throughout the breast, generally in favour of a benign pathology, such as inflammatory mastitis, rarely secondary to diffuse tumour infiltration such as lymphoma (figs. 61 and 62).

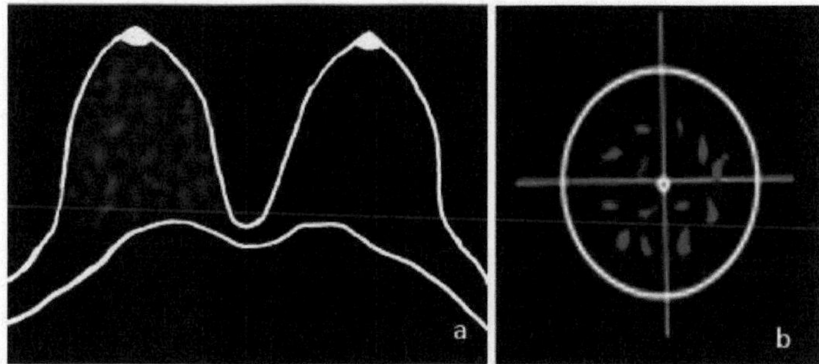

Fig. 61. Diagrams, diffuse non-mass enhancement (a+b).

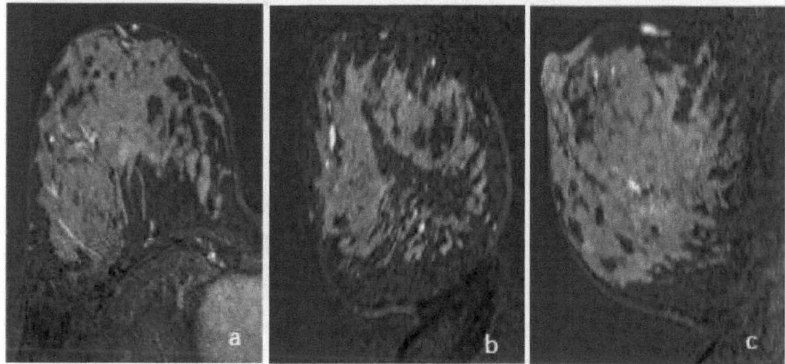

Fig. 62. Diffuse non-mass enhancement. Subtracted injected sequences, axial section (a), coronal section (b) and sagittal section (c). Non-mass enhancement evenly distributed throughout the breast.

- Bilateral diffuse non-mass enhancement and symmetrical

Bilateral enhancement and symmetry is a strong argument for benignity (fig. 63). The two main aetiologies responsible for this type of enhancement are physiological glandular enhancement and fibrocystic mastopathy, which most often results in micropunctate enhancement associated with microcysts visible on T2 (fig. 64).

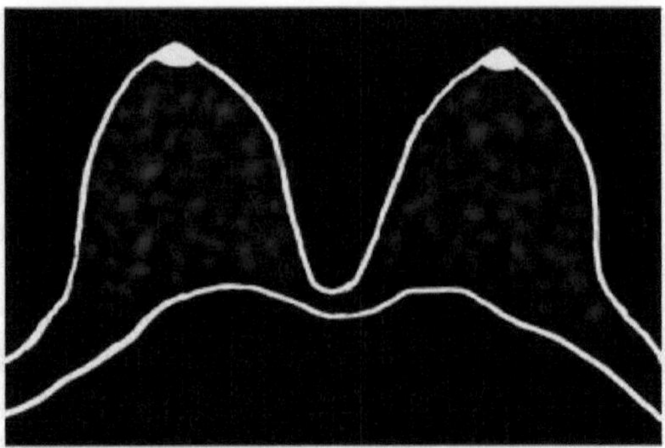

Fig. 63. Schematic diagram, bilateral and symmetrical diffuse non-mass enhancement.

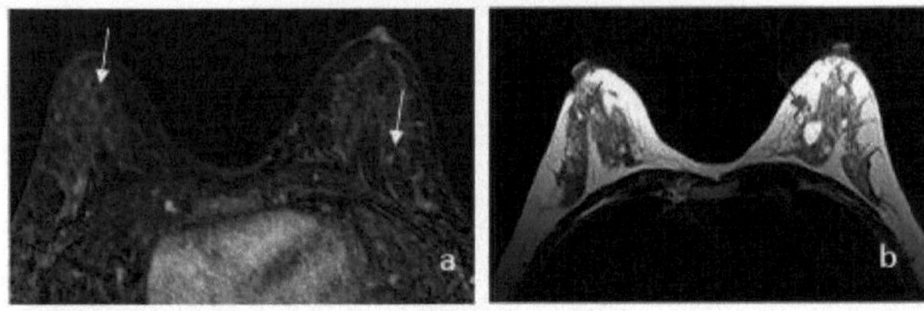

Fig. 64. Bilateral and symmetrical diffuse non-mass enhancement. Sequences injected subtraction, axial section (a), T2-weighted sequence (b). Non-mass enhancement of the micropunctate type on the injected sequences with the presence of a cyst in T2 hypersignal (arrows).

5.1.3.2 Raising characteristics

- ## Non-homogenous mass enhancement

Homogeneous enhancement is a confluent, uniform enhancement (figs. 65 and 66).

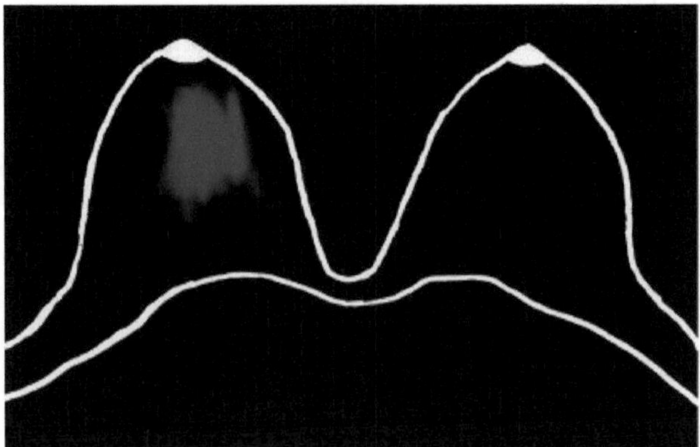

Fig. 65. Diagram, non-homogeneous mass enhancement.

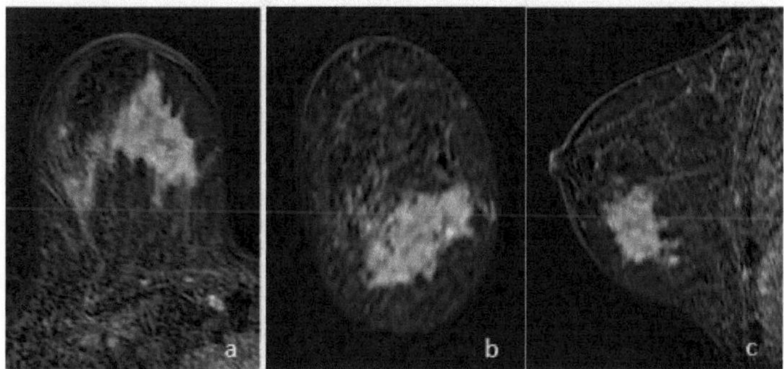

Fig. 66. Non-homogeneous mass enhancement. Subtracted injected sequences, axial section (a), coronal section (b) and sagittal section (c).

- ## Non-mass heterogeneous enhancement

Heterogeneous enhancement is non-uniform enhancement separated by areas of normal fat or glandular tissue [74] (figs. 67 and 68).

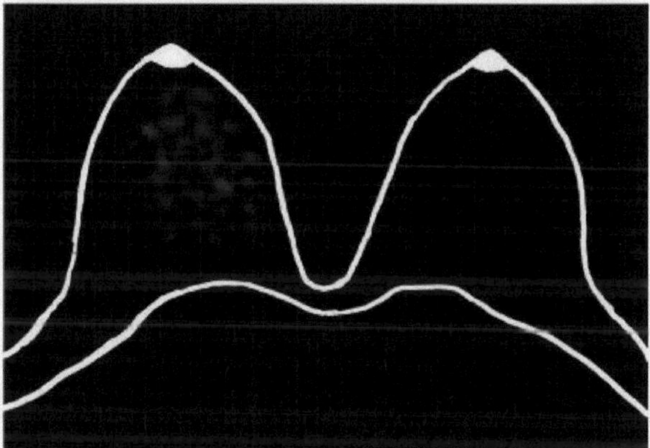

Fig. 67. Diagram, enhancement without heterogeneous mass.

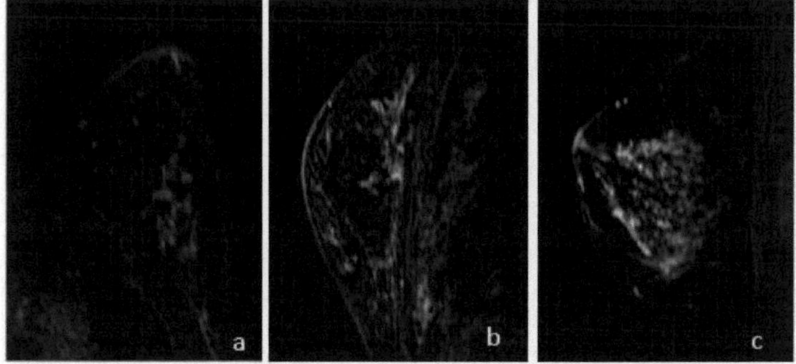

Fig. 68. Enhancement without heterogeneous mass. Subtracted injected

sequences, axial section (a) and sagittal sections (b+c).

• Non-micronodular enhancement

Micronodular enhancement corresponds to a grouping of small enhancements without masses or foci, often confluent in appearance (figs. 69 and 70).

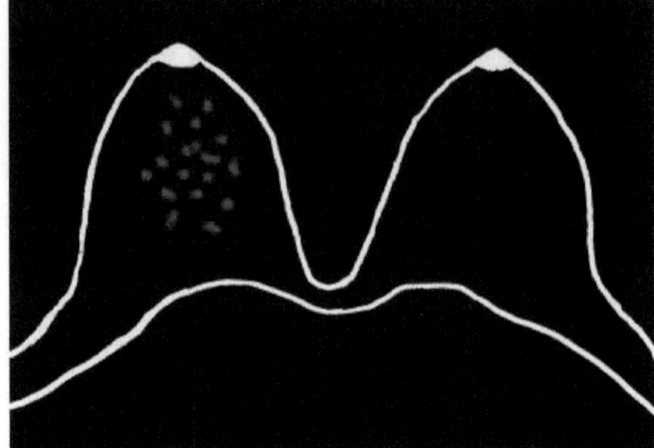

Fig. 69. Diagram, enhancement without micronodular mass.

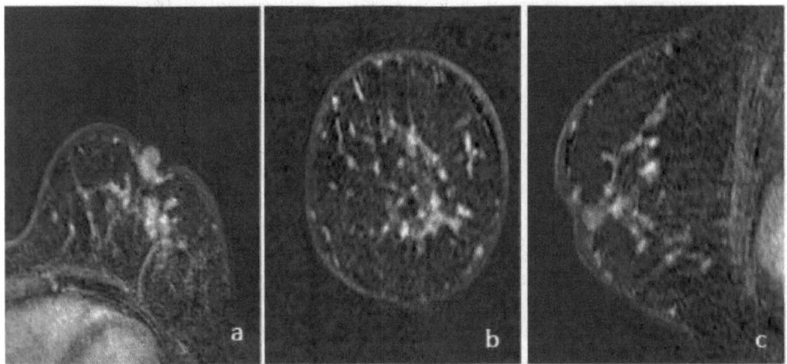

Fig. 70. Non-micronodular mass enhancement. Subtracted injected sequences, axial section (a), coronal section (b) and sagittal section (c).

• Non-ring mass cluster enhancement

Multiple confluent non-mass ring enhancements [73] (figs. 71 and 72).

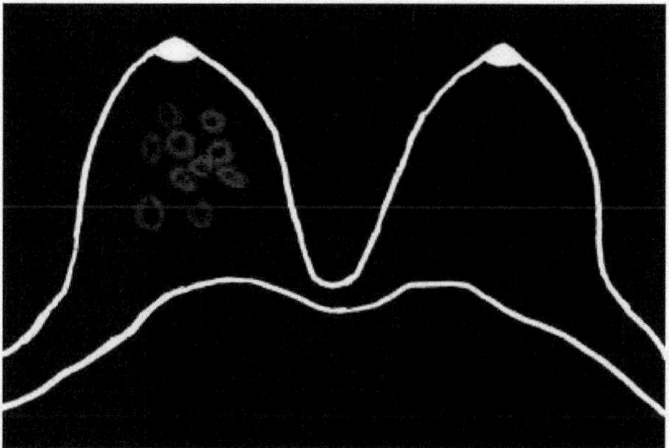

Fig. 71. Diagram, non-annular mass enhancement in a cluster.

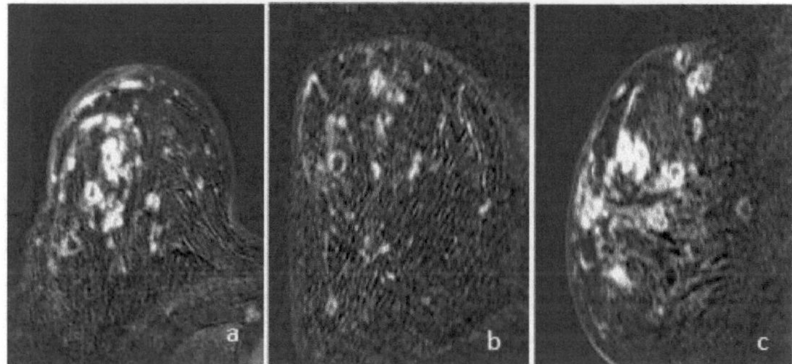

Fig. 72. Non-annular mass enhancement. Subtracted injected sequences, axial section (a), coronal section (b) and sagittal section (c).

5.2. Dynamic enhancement analysis

Analysis of the kinetics of enhancement will allow quantification of the intensity of enhancement of a lesion over time. Three types of curve have been defined by Kuhl et al [75] with analysis of the 2 parts of the curve: the initial part of the curve corresponds to the intensity of the signal during the 2 minutes following injection and the 2nd part of the curve corresponds to the intensity of the signal after the 2 minutes or when the curve bends.

5.2.1. Early phase enhancement

The intensity of enhancement is determined by the percentage of signal intensity of the lesion in the first two minutes after injection of the contrast agent.

- No raising

A signal increase of less than 2% after contrast injections (fig.73). The absence of enhancement is a very strong indicator of benignity such as fibrous scarring, fibroadenoma or cytosteatonecrosis. However, the absence of enhancement can be seen in malignant lesions after chemotherapy.

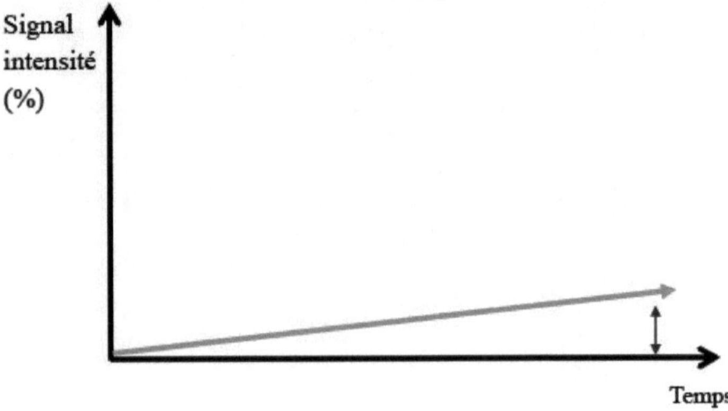

Fig. 73. No enhancement. Signal intensity less than 2% after 5 minutes.

- Slow raising

A maximum increase in signal intensity of less than 50% in the first 90 seconds after injection of contrast medium (fig. 74).

Slow initial enhancement is usually seen in fibrous fibroadenomas, adenoses and fibrous scarring. Rarely, carcinomas in situ may also show this type of enhancement probably due to recent chemotherapy or injection of insufficient contrast medium.

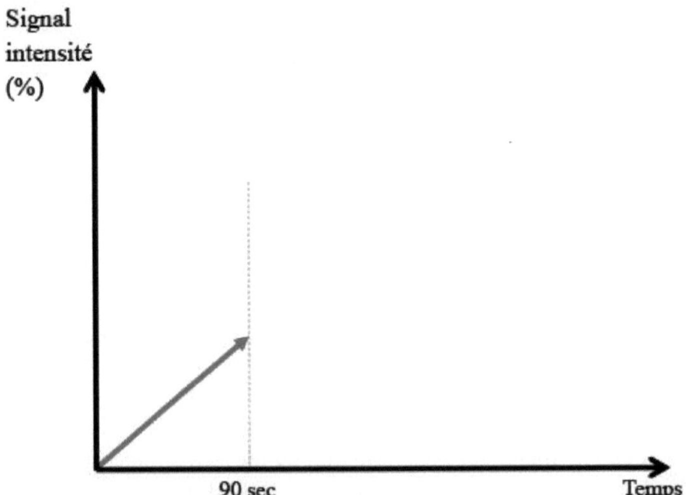

Fig. 74. Slow enhancement. Signal intensity less than 50% after the first 90 sec.

- Moderate raising

A 50% to 90% increase in signal intensity in the first 90 seconds after contrast injection (fig. 75). Moderate enhancement at the initial time is often seen in fibroadenomas and papillomas. Less frequently, this enhancement may occur in malignant lesions following chemotherapy.

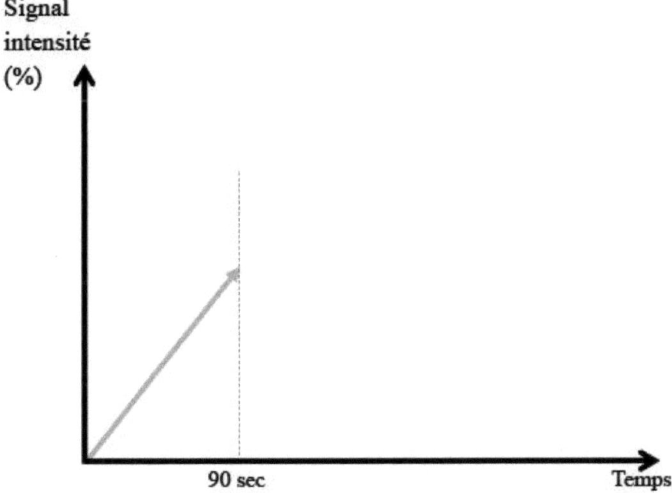

Fig. 75. Moderate enhancement. Signal intensity between 50% and 90% after the first 90 sec.

Quick lift

Maximum signal enhancement of over 90% occurs within 90 seconds of contrast injection (fig. 76). Initial rapid enhancement is often seen in invasive carcinomas. This enhancement may be observed rarely in intra mammary lymph nodes and myxoid fibroadenomas.

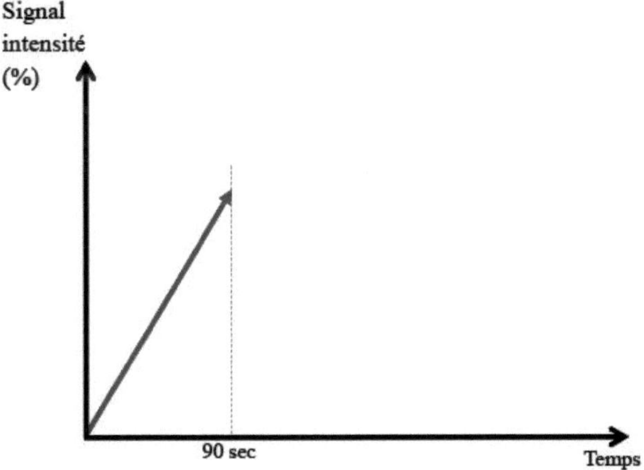

Fig. 76. Rapid enhancement. Signal intensity greater than 90% after the first 90 sec. Late phase enhancement

The intensity of enhancement is determined by the percentage of signal intensity of the lesion two minutes after injection of the contrast agent or when the curve bends.

- ## Persistent signal

Signal intensity continues to increase 2 minutes after contrast injection (fig. 77). Persistent enhancement is generally seen in benign masses such as myoid fibroadenoma or papilloma. In malignant lesions this type of signal is seen in only 10% of carcinomas, often infiltrating lobular carcinomas or foci of non-specific in situ carcinomas.

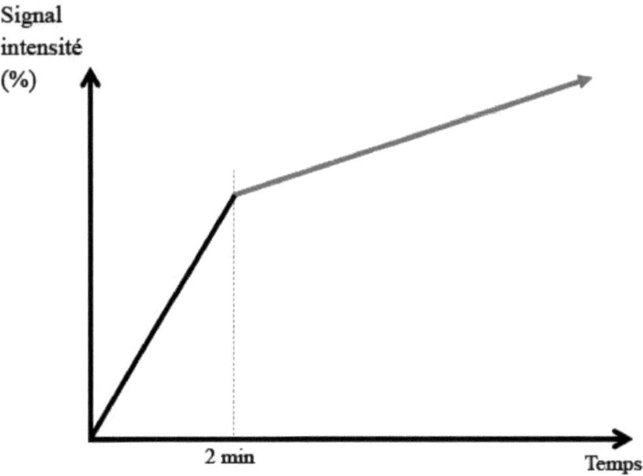

Fig. 77. Persistent signal. Signal intensity continues to increase after 2 minutes.

- ## Signal on set

The signal intensity remains constant after the maximum peak (fig. 78). This type of signal is particularly common in papillomas.

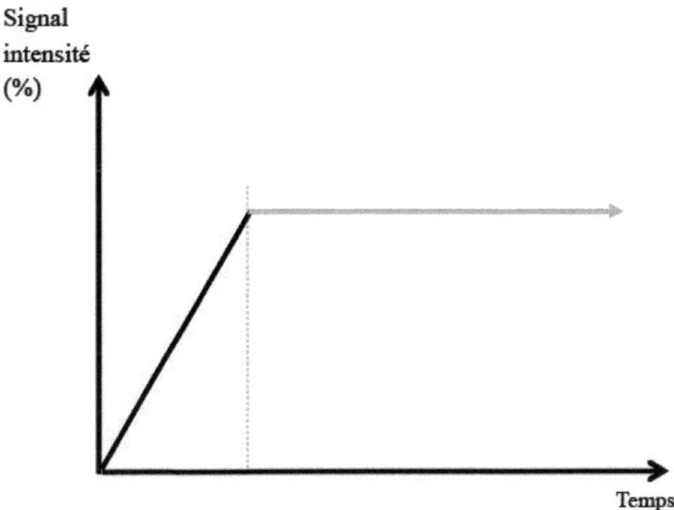

Fig. 78. Signal plateau. Signal intensity remains constant after the maximum peak.

Washing out the signal

Washout is defined as a fall in signal of more than 10% after the maximum intensity at the initial time, and is the main dynamic criterion of a malignant lesion (fig. 79). This rapid washout of contrast medium in a malignant lesion is probably caused by the arteriovenous shunts of intratumoral angiogenesis. Washing is rarely seen in benign pathologies.

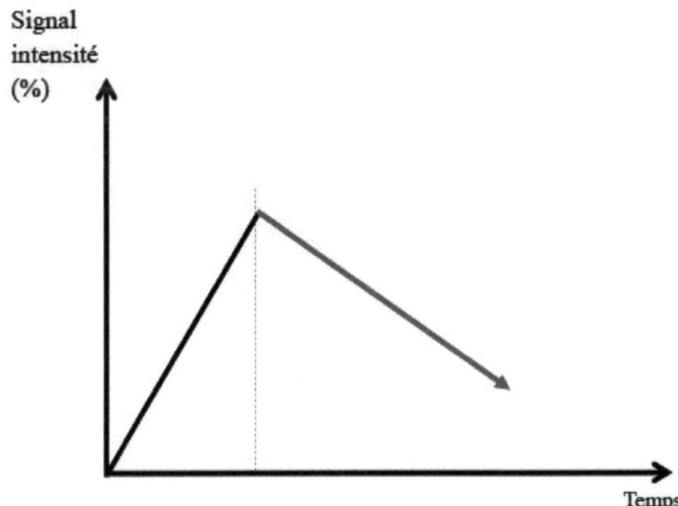

Fig. 79. Signal washout. Signal intensity drops by more than 10% after the

maximum peak.

5.2.2. Classification of enhancement curves

The three types of enhancement curves described by CK. Kuhl et al [75]:

- Type I: an initial slow, then progressive, enhancement curve (fig. 80)
- Type II: a rapid initial enhancement curve, followed by a plateau (fig. 81).
- Type III: a rapid initial enhancement curve, followed by a washout (fig. 82).

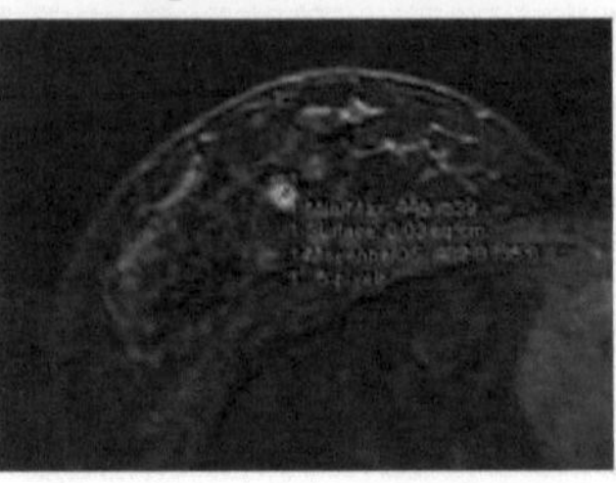
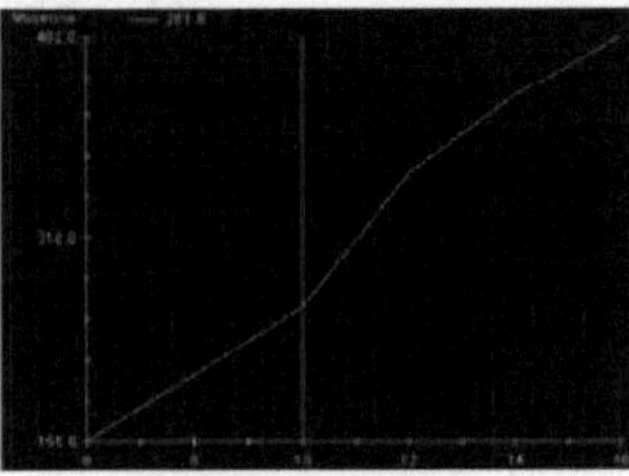

Fig. 80. Type I curve. Subtracted injected sequences, axial section (a) and enhancement curve (b). Histology: fibroadenoma.

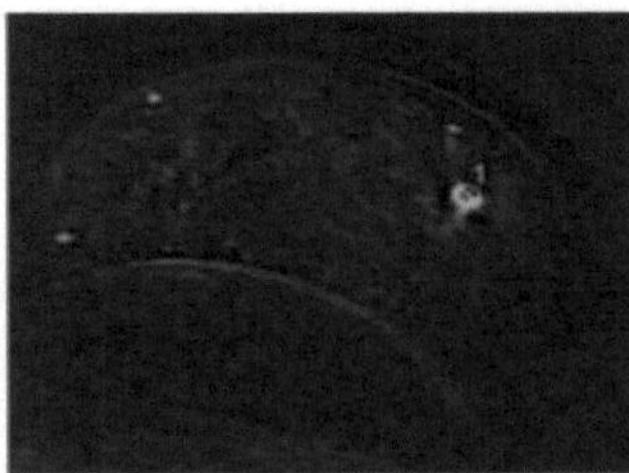
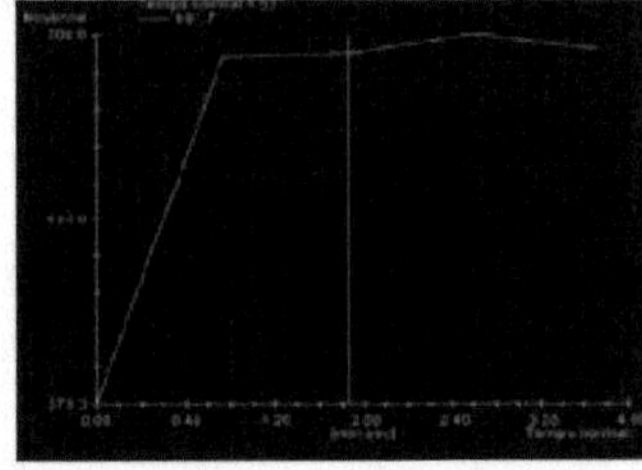

Fig. 81. Type II curve. Subtracted injected sequences, axial section (a) and enhancement curve (b). Histology: fibroadenoma.

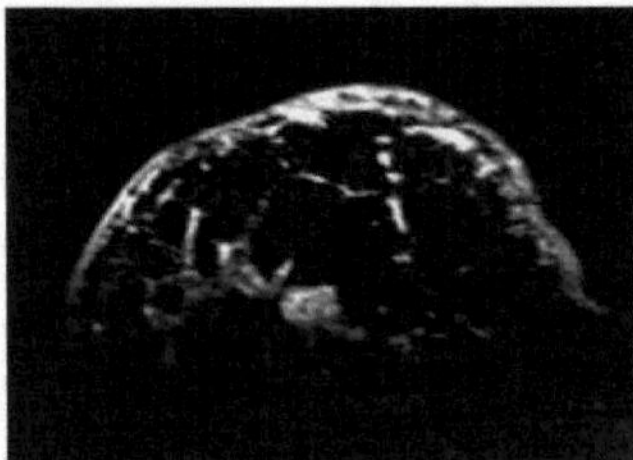
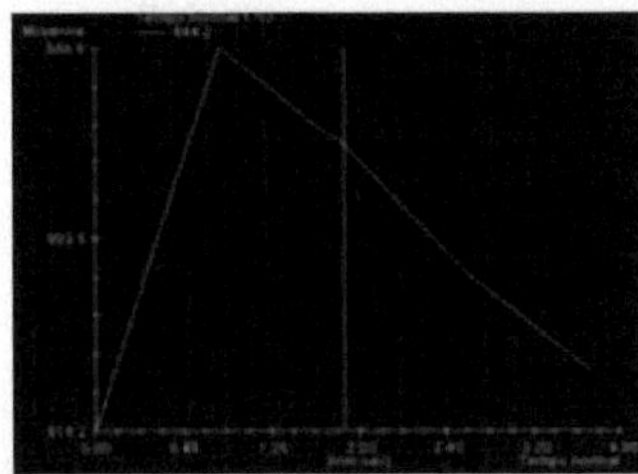

Fig. 82. Type III curve. Subtracted injected sequences, axial section (a) and enhancement curve (b). Histology: Invasive lobular carcinoma.

5.3 Other signs on breast MRI

- Hook sign

The hook sign is a thin line running from the lesion to the pectoral muscle, with little or no enhancement after injection of contrast (Fig. 83). The hook sign may be secondary to a desmoplastic reaction or peritumoral carcinomatous lymphangitis (fig. 84) [76, 77]. The hook sign can also be seen in the post-operative scar, presenting as a thin fibrous line, unenhanced after injection of contrast (Fig. 85).

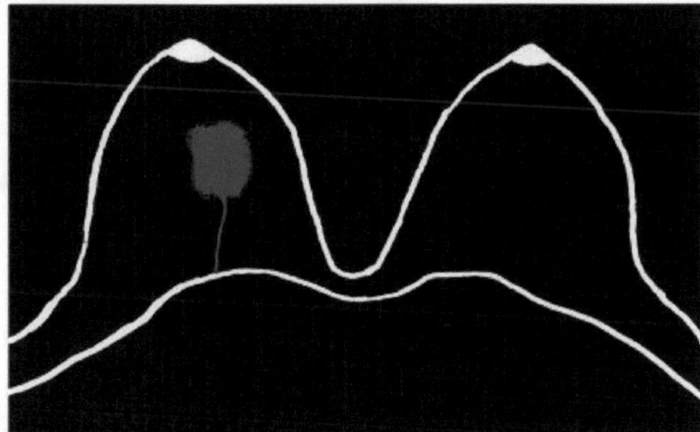

Fig. 83. Hook sign, diagram.

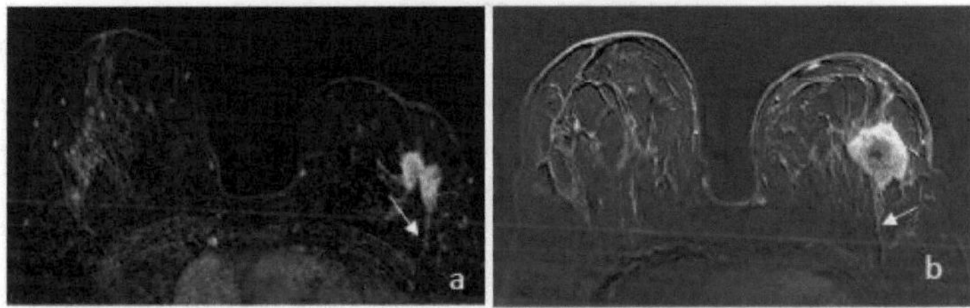

Fig. 84. Hook sign secondary to a desmoplastic reaction. Sequences subtracted injected (a+b). Masses of irregular shape and contours, with heterogeneous enhancement and the presence of a thin line running from the mass to the pectoral muscle, enhanced after injection of contrast medium (arrows).

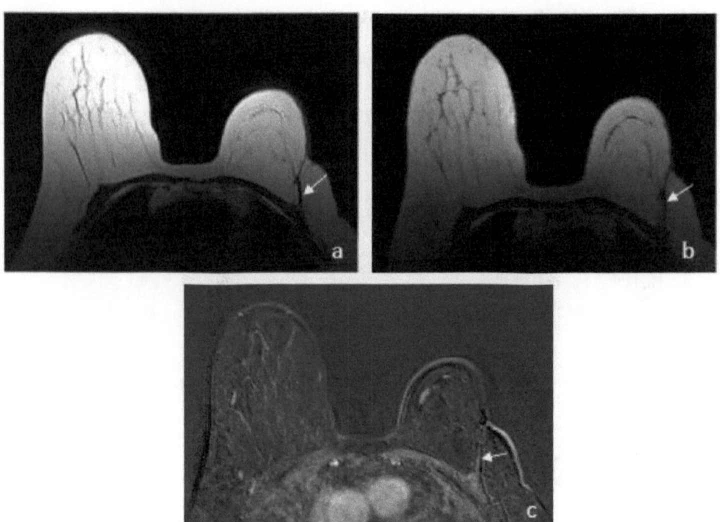

Fig. 85. Postoperative hook sign. T2-weighted sequence (a), T1-weighted sequence (b) and injected subtraction sequence (c). Thin fibrous postoperative line running from the cutaneous plane to the pectoral muscle, unenhanced after injection of contrast medium (arrows).

- (Perifocal edema

A redematous ring, complete or incomplete around the lesion (fig. 86). This peri-lesional redema is suggestive of a malignant lesion with a poor prognosis. It may be secondary to increased activity of the tumour's angiogenic enzymes [78] (fig. 87)

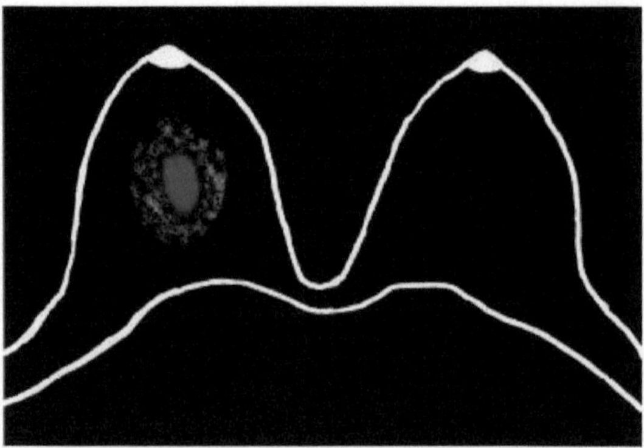

Fig. 86. Perifocal oedema, diagram.

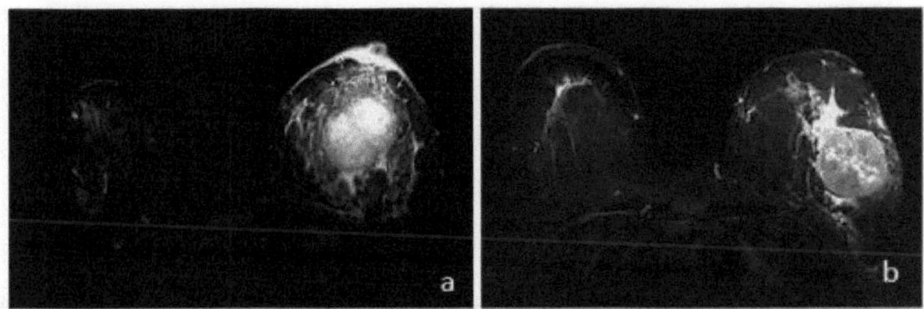

Fig. 87. Perifocal oedema. Fat Sat T2-weighted sequences (a+b). Masses of irregular shape and contour, surrounded by peri-lesional oedema (arrows).

- Sign of the eclipse

Raising of the cystic wall resembling a solar eclipse, found in inflammatory cysts (figs. 88 and 89).

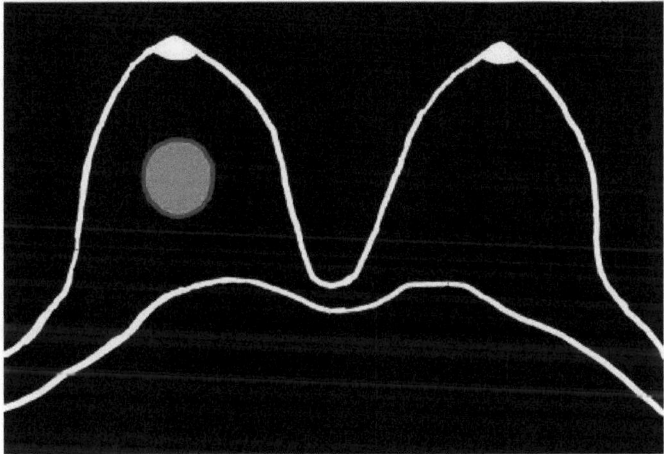

Fig. 88. Eclipse sign, diagram.

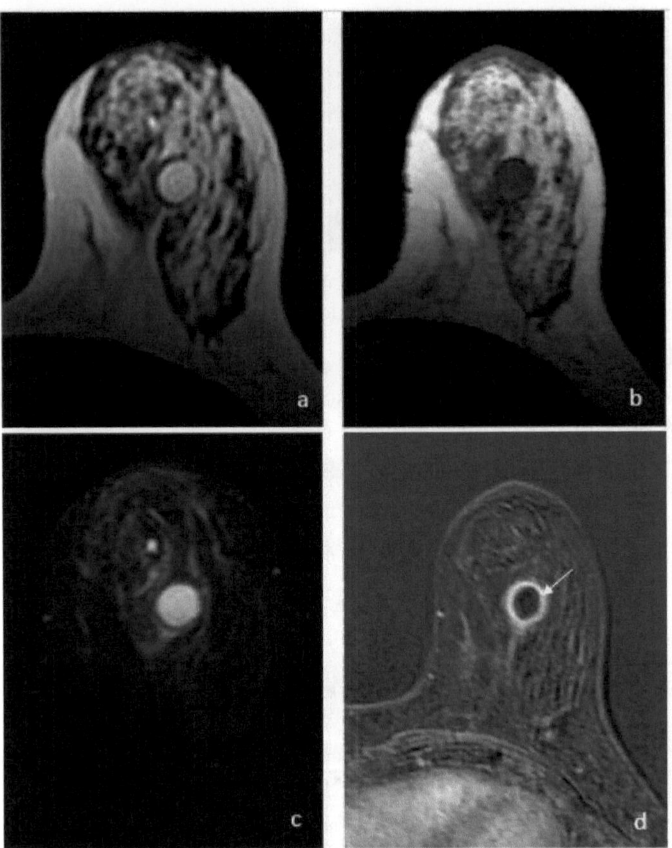

Fig. 89. Eclipse sign. T2-weighted sequence (a), T1-weighted sequence (b), T2 Fat Sat-weighted sequence (c) and injected subtraction sequence (d). Round lesion with circumscribed contours, hypersignal T2 and T2 Fat Sat, hyposignal T1, thickened wall hyposignal T1 and T2, enhanced after injection of contrast product resembling a solar eclipse (arrow). Histology: inflammatory cyst.

Invasion of the pectoral muscle

Invasion of the pectoral muscle is seen in the form of enhancement extending from the malignant mass to the pectoral muscle (figs. 90 and 91).

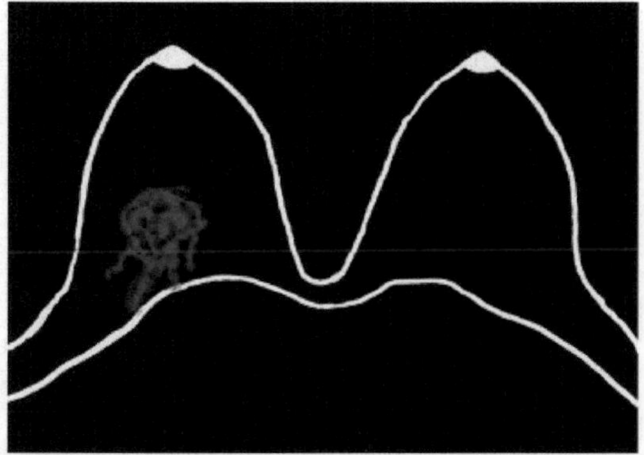

Fig. 90. Invasion of the pectoralis muscle, diagram.

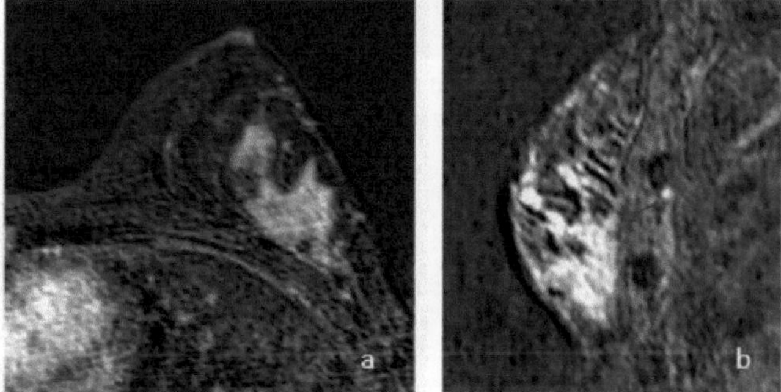

Fig. 91. Invasion of the pectoralis muscle. Subtracted sequences injected, Axial section (a) and sagittal section (b). Extension to the pectoralis muscle (arrows).

- Nipple retraction

The nipple is retracted into the retroareolar tissue (Fig. 92). Nipple retraction is particularly suspicious in cases of unilateral nipple enhancement (Fig. 93). A non-enhanced retracted nipple may be related to a variant of normal or secondary to mastitis, surgery or irradiation.

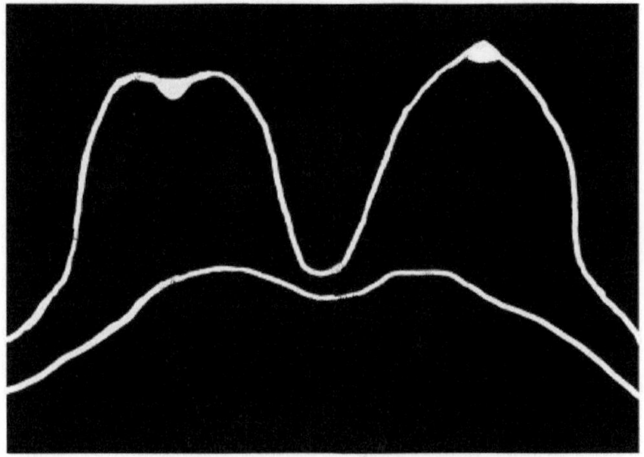

Fig. 92. Nipple retraction, diagram.

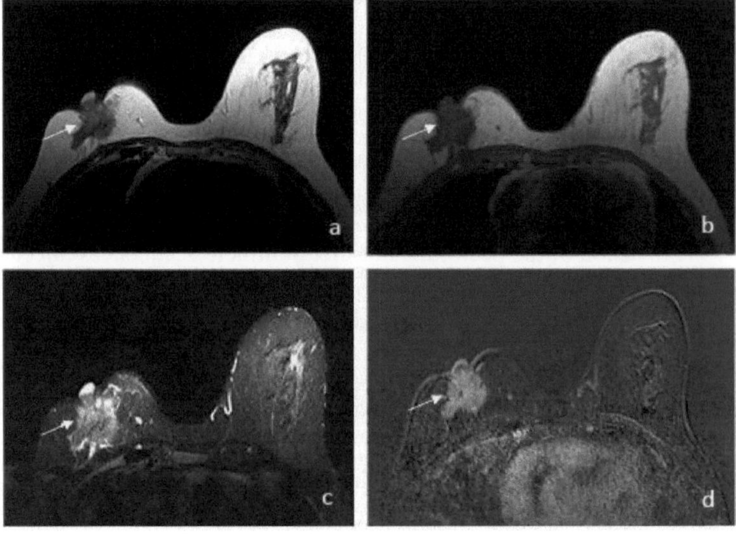

Fig. 93. Nipple retraction. T2-weighted sequence (a), T1-weighted sequence (b), T2 Fat Sat-weighted sequence (c) and injected subtraction sequence (d). A mass of irregular shape and contours, in T1, T2 and T2 Fat Sat hypopositivity, with heterogeneous enhancement after injection of contrast product, retracting the nipple (arrows). Histology: non-specific infiltrating carcinoma.

- Skin retraction

Cutaneous retraction is a fold in the skin and is a classic sign of malignant lesions, often associated with fine lines enhanced after injection of contrast medium between the malignant mass and the skin covering (figs. 94 and 95).

Skin retraction can also occur after surgery or radiotherapy (figs. 96 and 97).

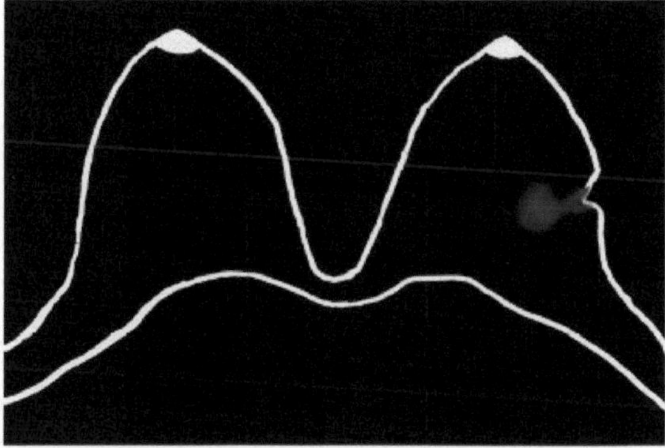

Fig. 94. Skin retraction secondary to a malignant mass, diagram.

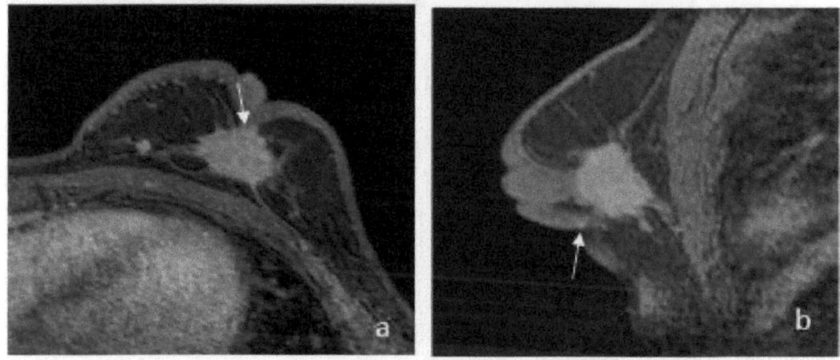

Fig. 95. Cutaneous retraction secondary to a malignant lesion. Subtracted injected sequences, axial section (a) and sagittal section (b).

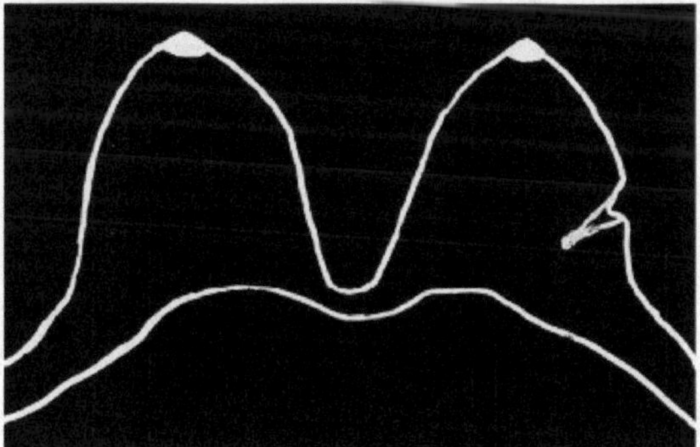

Fig. 96. Postoperative skin retraction, diagram.

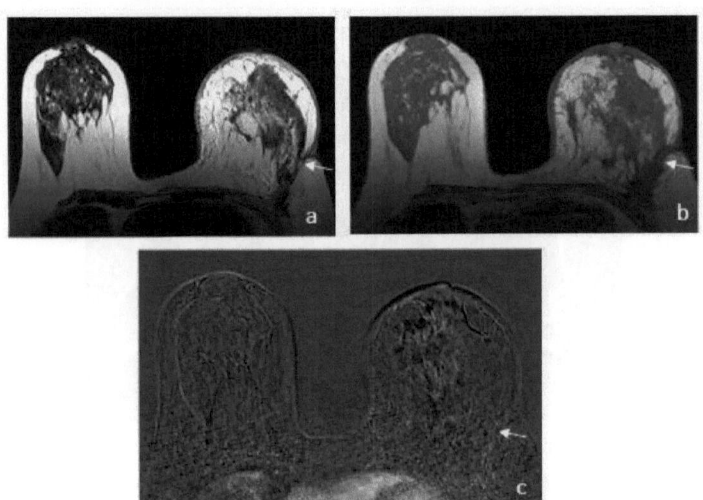

Fig. 97. Postoperative skin retraction. T2-weighted sequence (a), T1-weighted sequence (b) and injected subtraction sequence (c). Postoperative skin retraction in T1, T2 hyposignal, unenhanced after injection of contrast medium (arrows).

- Unilateral diffuse skin thickening

The skin layer is thicker than that of the contralateral breast (Fig. 98). This diffuse thickening is a frequent consequence of surgery, radiotherapy or previous mastitis [79] (fig. 99). It may also be observed in carcinomatous mastitis associated with other signs of malignancy such as a mass, non-mass enhancement and redema [80] (fig. 100).

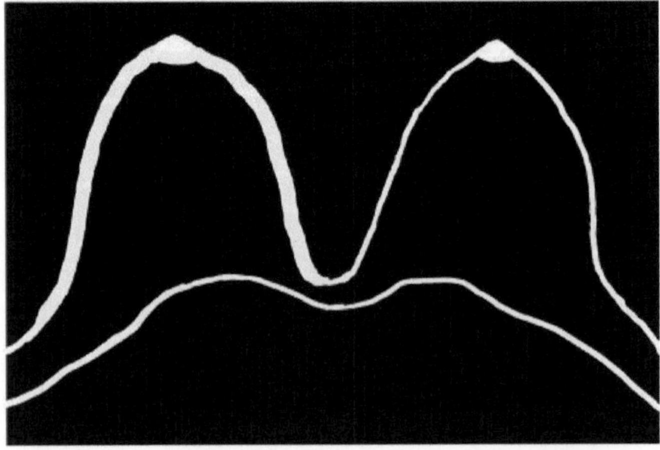

Fig. 98. Unilateral diffuse skin thickening, diagram.

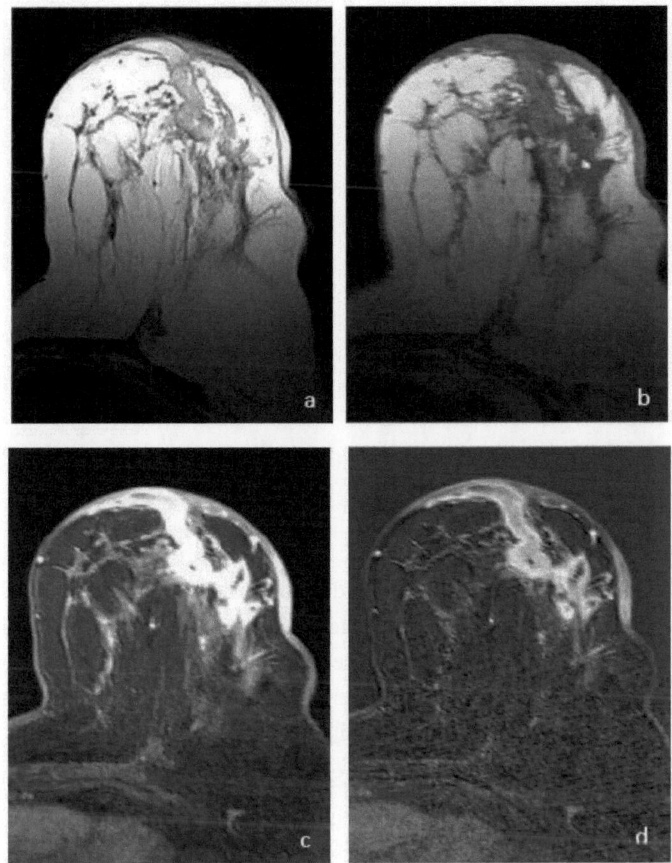

Fig. 99. Unilateral diffuse skin thickening secondary to a malignant lesion. T2-weighted sequence (a), T1-weighted sequence (b), native injected T1 sequence (c) and subtracted injected sequence (d). Diffuse skin thickening in T2 and T1 hyposignal, enhanced after injection of contrast medium secondary to a malignant mass.

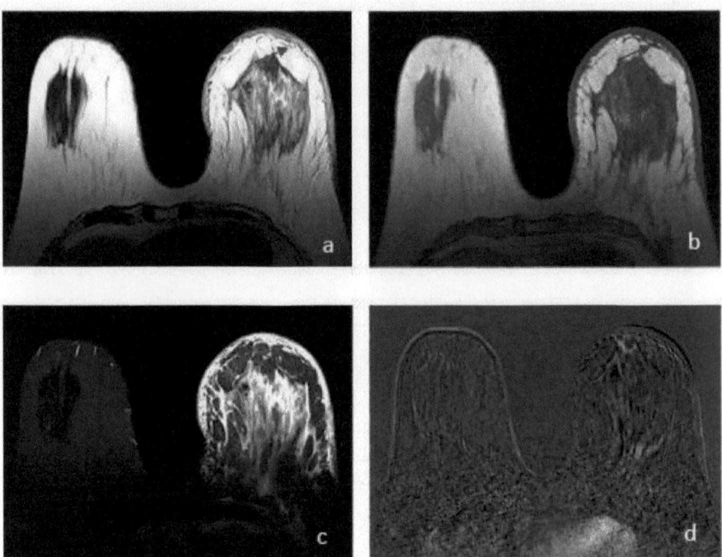

Fig. 100. Nipple retraction secondary to radiotherapy. Sequence in T2-weighted sequence (a), T1-weighted sequence (b), T2 Fat Sat-weighted sequence (c) and injected subtraction sequence (d). Diffuse skin thickening in T2 and T1 hyposignal, T2 Fat Sat hypersignal, not enhanced after injection of secondary contrast (arrows).

- Increased subcutaneous vascularisation

The presence of subcutaneous vascularisation is often secondary to surgery or radiotherapy (figs. 101 and 102). Increased subcutaneous vascularisation can be seen in breast carcinomas, but exceptionally as an isolated sign (fig. 103). Vascular thrombosis in the contralateral breast (internal mammary artery and vein or lateral thoracic artery and vein) is also possible but very rare.

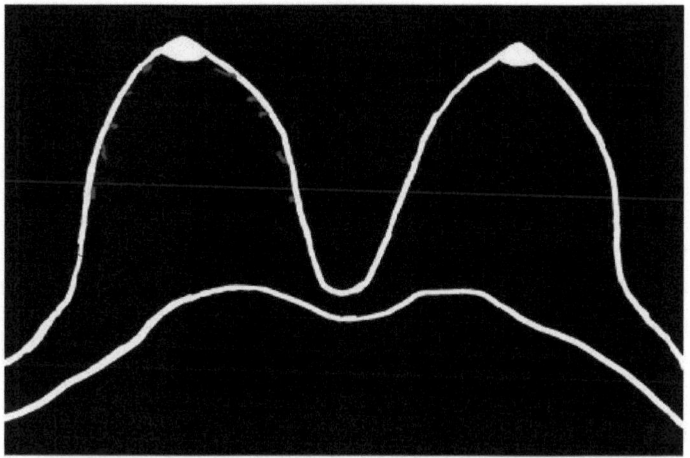

Fig. 101. Increase in subcutaneous vascularisation, diagram.

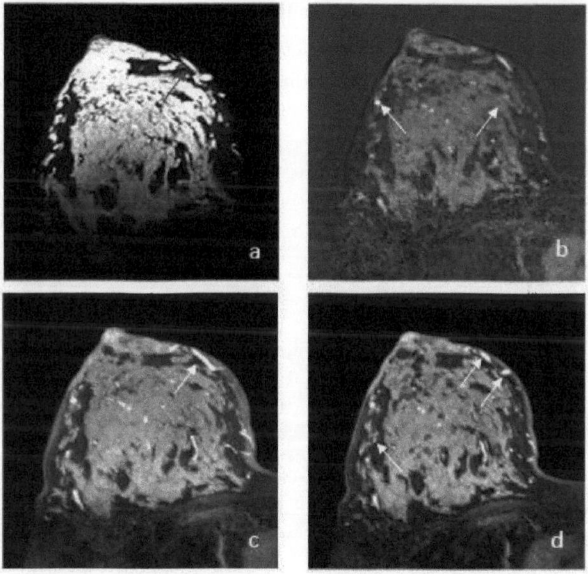

Fig. 102. Post-radiation increase in subcutaneous vascularisation. Fat Sat T2-weighted sequence (a), injected subtraction sequence (b) and native injected T1 sequence (c + d). Increased subcutaneous vascularisation associated with oedema of the fibro-glandular framework in post-radiation T2 Fat Sat hypersignal (arrows).

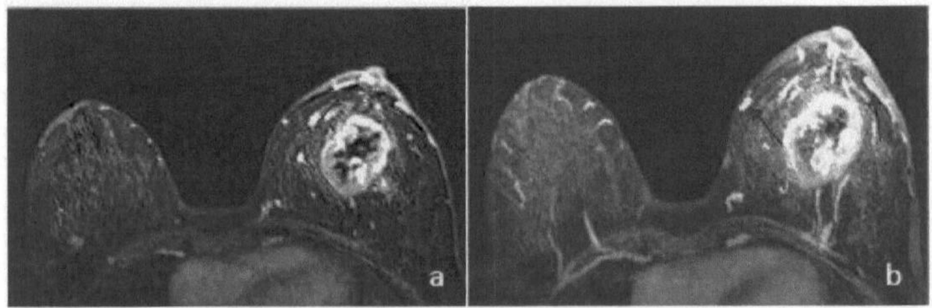

Fig. 103. Increase in subcutaneous vascularisation secondary to a malignant lesion. Injected subtraction sequence (a), MIP reconstruction (b). Increased subcutaneous vascularisation associated with a malignant mass with annular enhancement (arrows).

- (Subcutaneous edema

Redness in the subcutaneous region, best appreciated on STIR or TSE T2 images (fig. 104). This swelling may be the result of radiotherapy or inflammation [81, 82] (fig. 105). This is easily determined from the patient's history. If radiotherapy and inflammation are ruled out, carcinomatous mastitis should be suspected.

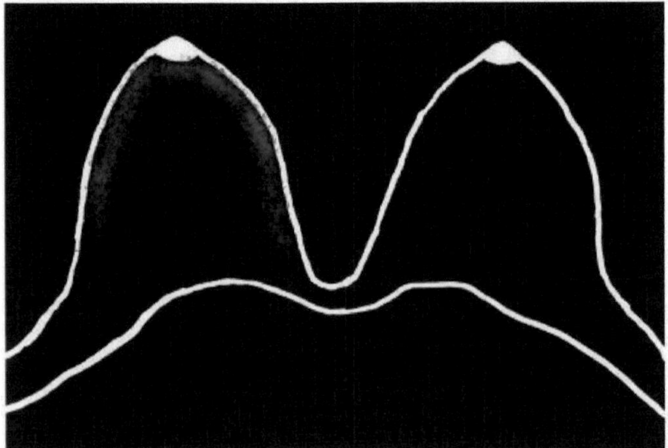

Fig. 104. Subcutaneous oedema, diagram.

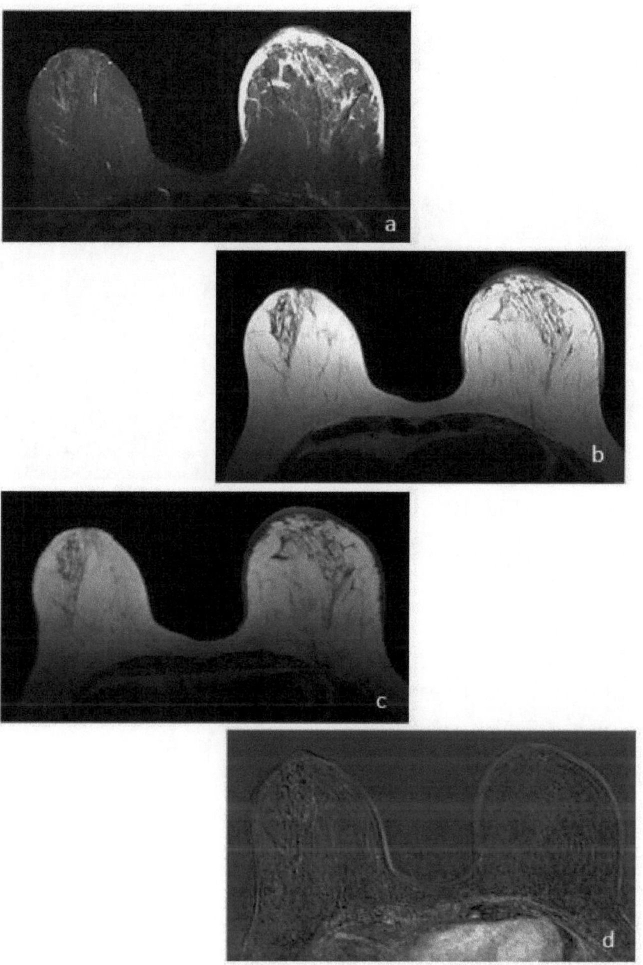

Fig. 105. Post-radiation subcutaneous oedema. Fat Sat T2-weighted sequence (a), T2-weighted sequence (b), T1-weighted sequence (c) and injected subtraction sequence (d). Subcutaneous oedema in T2 fat-sat hypersignal (arrows) associated with skin thickening, in T1 and T2 hyposignal, not enhanced post-radiation.

- (Unilateral edema

Presence of swelling in one breast, detectable on TSE T2 sequences or better on STIR images (fig. 106). Unilateral breast swelling is generally found in carcinomatous mastitis [83-87] (fig. 107). However, this sign is also present after surgery or radiotherapy. Swelling is particularly frequent after radiotherapy and may persist for several years [82, 85] (fig. 108).

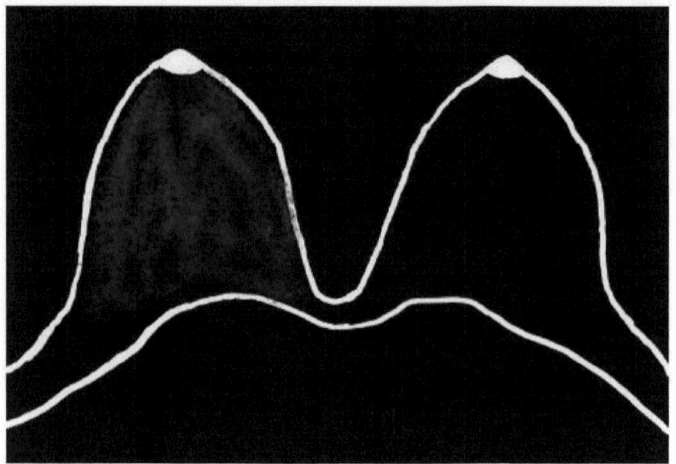

Fig. 106. Unilateral oedema, diagram.

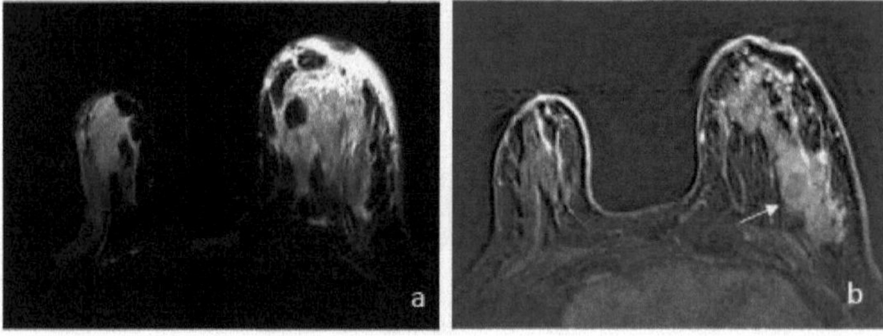

Fig. 107. Unilateral oedema secondary to a malignant lesion. Fat Sat T2-weighted sequence (a) and injected subtraction sequence (b). Left unilateral oedema with hypersignal T2 Fat Sat on the injected sequences, showing a mass suspicious of malignancy with irregular shape and contours and heterogeneous enhancement (arrow).

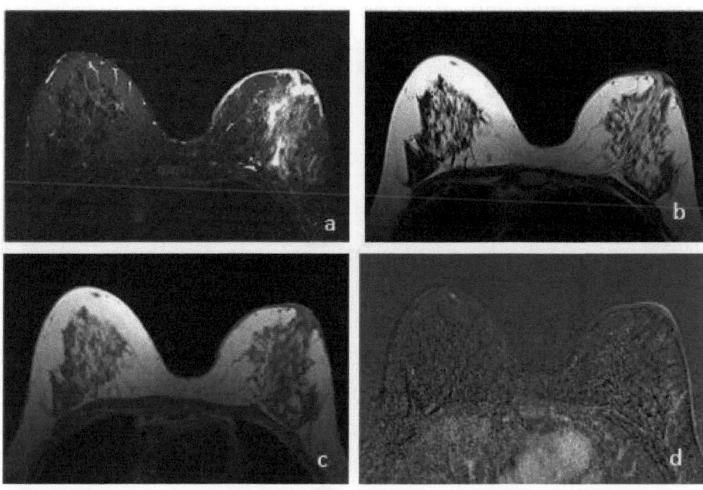

Fig. 108. Unilateral post-radiation oedema. Fat Sat T2-weighted sequence (a), T2-weighted sequence (b), T1-weighted sequence (c) and injected subtraction sequence (d). Left unilateral oedema with hypersignal T2 Fat Sat associated with skin thickening, with hyposignal T1 and T2 post-radiation.

(Prepectoral edema

Edema located in front of the pectoral muscle (fig. 109). Like all signs of swelling, this sign appears better on STIR sequences than on T2 TSE sequences (fig. 110). Prepectoral edema in an untreated breast is strongly suggestive of a malignant lesion. This is probably due to tumour invasion and increased activity of angiogenic enzymes along the pectoralis muscle [83, 84]. Other causes of prepectoral edema are surgery and radiotherapy [81, 82] (fig. 111).

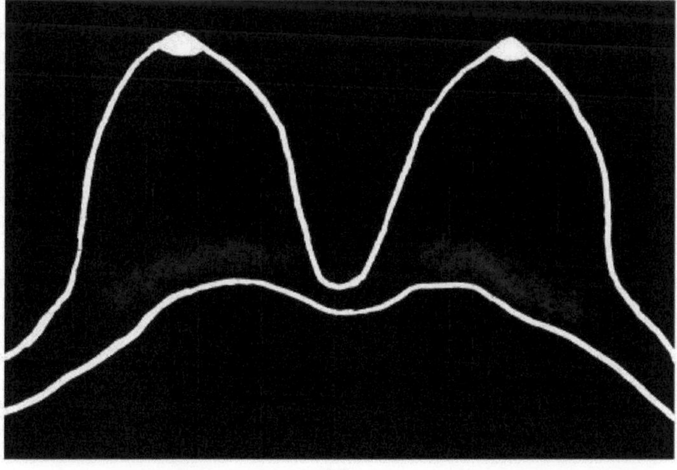

Fig. 109. Prepectoral oedema, diagram.

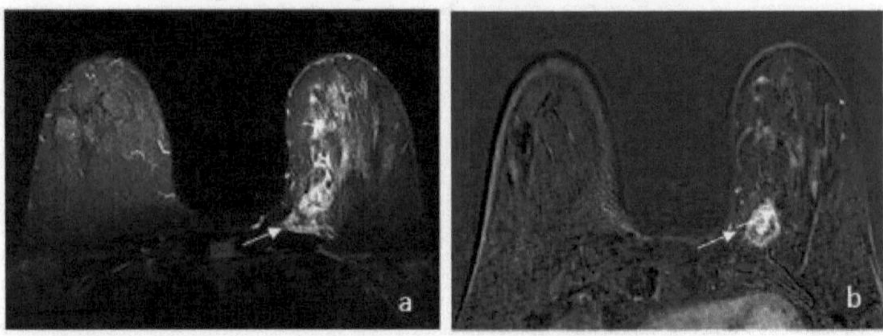

Fig. 110. Prepectoral oedema secondary to a malignant lesion. Fat Sat T2-weighted sequence (a) and injected subtraction sequence (b). Left prepectoral oedema with hypersignal T2 Fat Sat (arrow) associated with a mass suspicious of malignancy of irregular shape and contours, with heterogeneous enhancement (arrow).

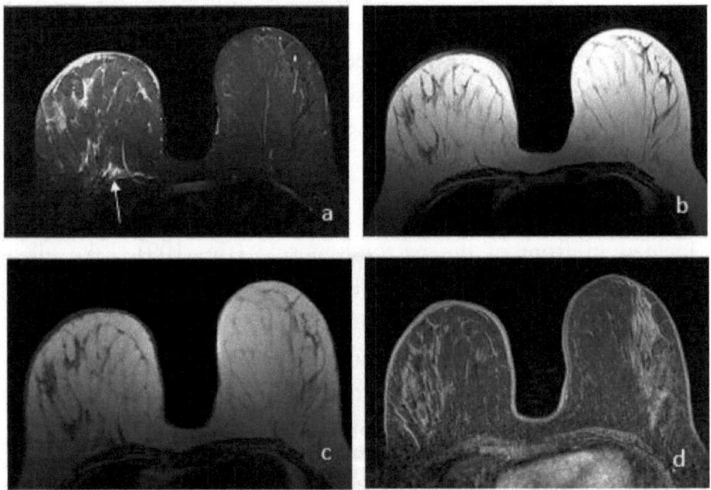

Fig. 111. Post-radiation prepectoral oedema. Fat Sat T2-weighted sequence (a), T2-weighted sequence (b), T1-weighted sequence (c) and injected subtraction sequence (d). Right prepectoral oedema in T2 fat-sat hypersignal (arrow), with no translation on T2, T1 and injected sequences.

Axillary adenopathy

Round or spherical lymph node, more than 1 cm in diameter, enhanced after injection of contrast medium (fig. 112). On T1 and T2 images, the hypersignal of the lymph node hilum disappears (fig. 113). These lymph nodes are generally of metastatic origin [88].

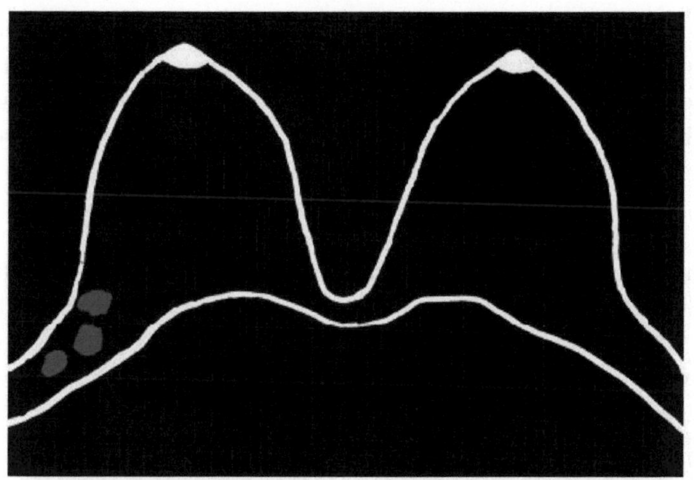

Fig. 112. Axillary adenopathy, diagram.

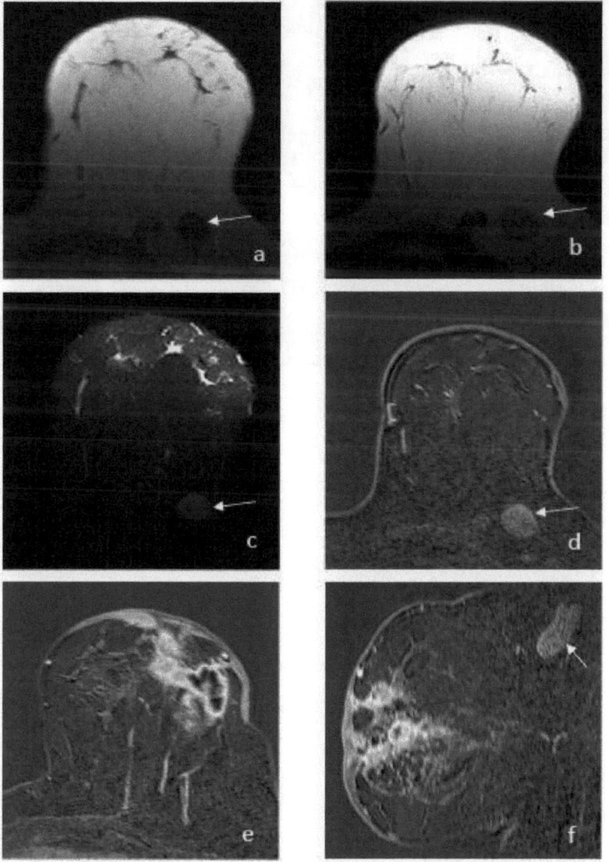

Fig. 113. Axillary adenopathy. T2-weighted sequence (a), T1-weighted sequence (b), T2 Fat Sat-weighted sequence (c) and injected subtraction sequence, axial sections (d+e), sagittal section (f). Axillary adenopathy with T1 and T2 hyposignal, T2 Fat Sat hypersignal, enhanced after injection of contrast medium (arrows) associated with a malignant mass of irregular shape and contours, with heterogeneous enhancement (red arrows).

The signal intensity of the lesion on T2-weighted sequences is less than the signal intensity of the surrounding normal parenchyma (fig. 114). A T2 low-intensity lesion may be associated with fibroadenoma, radial scarring or carcinoma, which generally presents with associated signs such as hook sign, perifocal lesion, etc [89-91] (figs. 115 and 116).

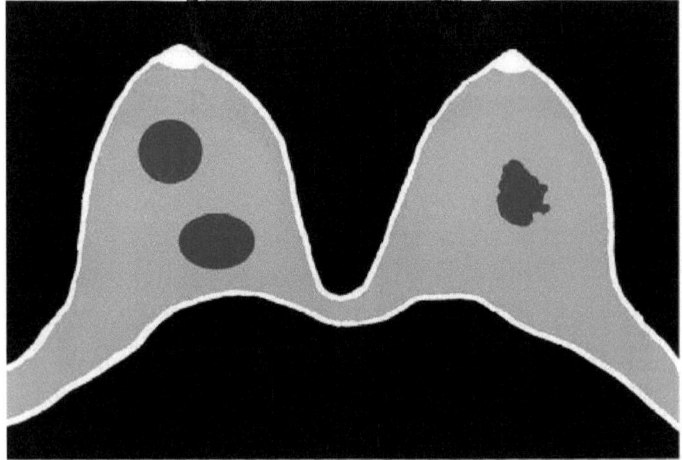

Fig. 114. Low-positivity T2 lesion, diagram.

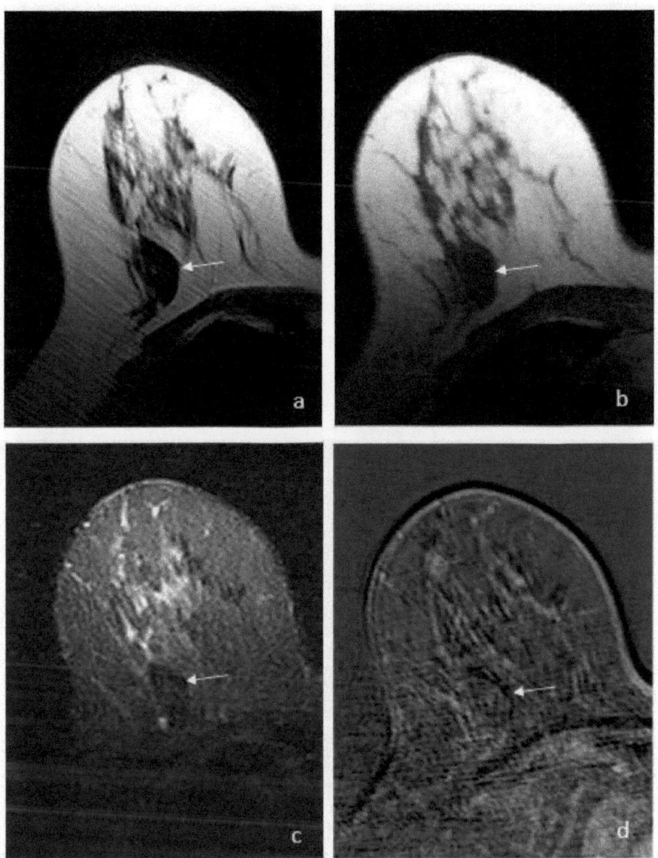

Fig. 115. T2-hyposignal mass. T2-weighted sequence (a), T1-weighted sequence (b), T2 Fat Sat-weighted sequence (c) and injected subtraction sequence (d). Oval mass, with circumscribed contours, in hyposignal T1, T2 and T2 Fat Sat, weakly enhanced after injection of contrast product on subtracted sequences (arrows). Histology: fibroadenoma.

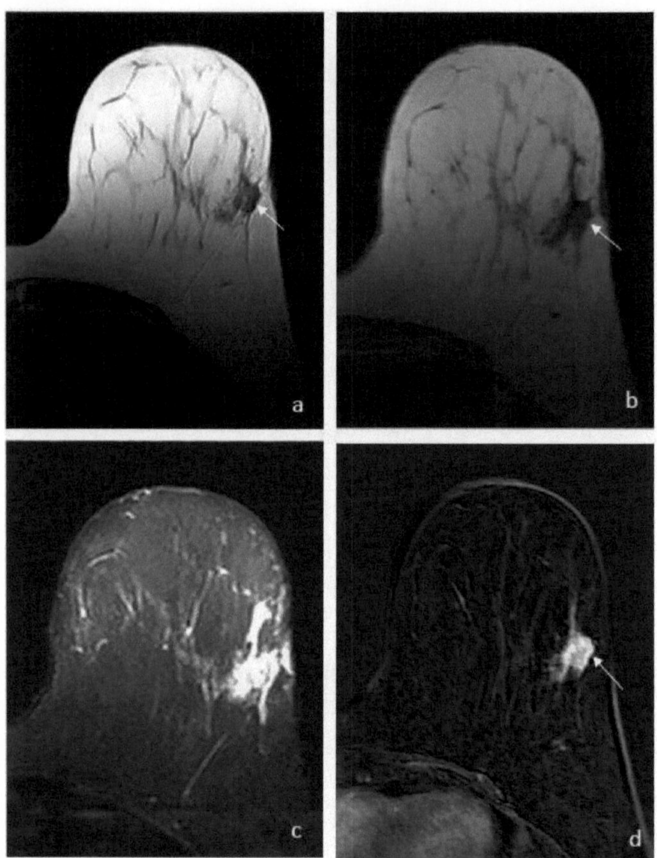

Fig. 116. Low T2 mass. T2-weighted sequence (a), T1-weighted sequence (b), T2 Fat Sat sequence (c) and injected subtraction sequence (d). Mass of irregular shape and contours, in T1 and T2 hypersignal, with heterogeneous enhancement on injected sequences (arrows) surrounded by peri-lesional oedema in T2 Fat Sat hypersignal (red arrow). Histology: non-specific infiltrating carcinoma.

The signal intensity of the lesion on T2-weighted sequences is equal to that of the surrounding normal parenchyma (fig. 117). Isointense signal is generally seen in fibrous fibroadenomas and rarely in myxoid fibroadenomas [91]. Malignant lesions may have an isointense signal but more often a hypointense T2 signal (Fig. 118).

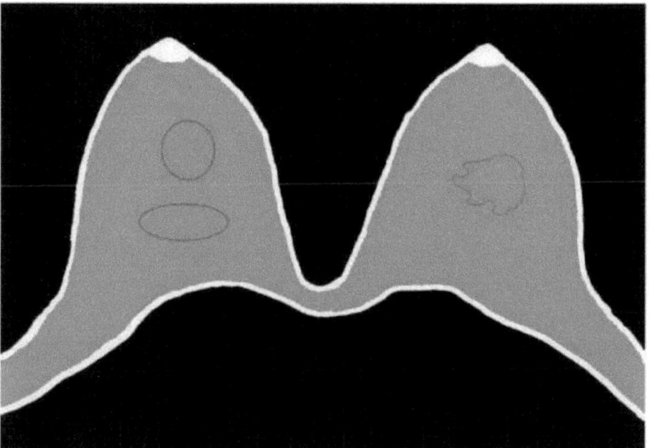

Fig. 117. T2 isosignal lesion, diagram.

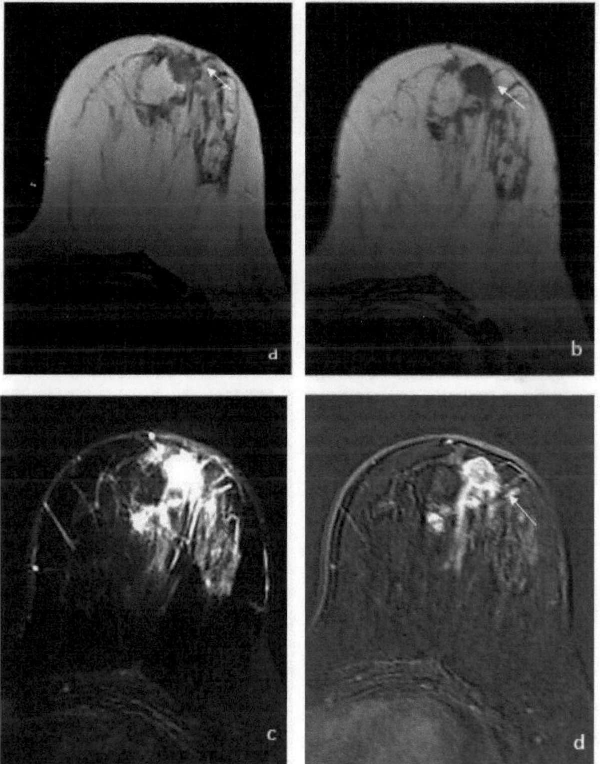

Fig. 118. Low T2 mass. T2-weighted sequence (a), T1-weighted sequence (b), T2 Fat Sat sequence (c) and injected subtraction sequence (d). Mass of irregular shape and contours, T2 isosignal to normal parenchyma, T1 hyposignal, heterogeneously enhanced on injected sequences (arrows) surrounded by peri-lesional oedema in T2 Fat Sat hypersignal (red arrow). Histology: non-specific infiltrating carcinoma.

- T2 hypersignal

The signal intensity of the lesion on T2-weighted sequences is greater than the signal intensity of the surrounding normal parenchyma (fig. 119). T2 hypersignal is found in cysts, the signal intensity of which varies according to the fluid content. T2 hypersignal may also be found in fatty cytosteonecrosis and mucinous fibroadenomas, where the mucinous mesenchymal component is responsible for the high signal (figs 120 and 121). Malignant lesions may be T2 hyperintense [92] (fig. 122).

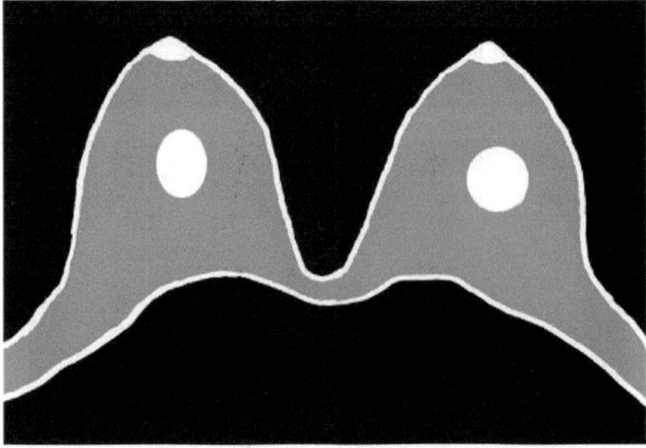

Fig. 119. T2 hypersignal lesion, diagram.

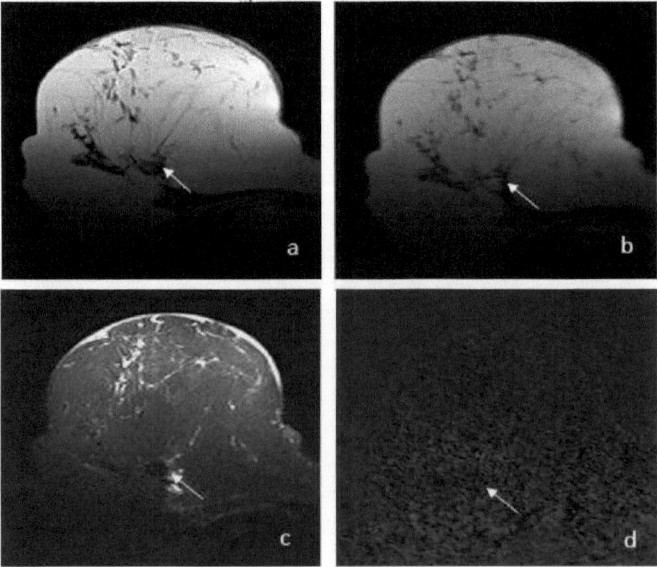

Fig. 120. T2 hypersignal lesion. T2-weighted sequence (a), T1-weighted sequence (b), T2 Fat Sat-weighted sequence (c) and injected subtraction sequence (d). Oval lesion with irregular contours, hypersignal T1, T2, hyposignal T2 Fat Sat, not enhanced after injection of contrast product on subtraction sequences (arrows). Histology: cytosteatonecrosis.

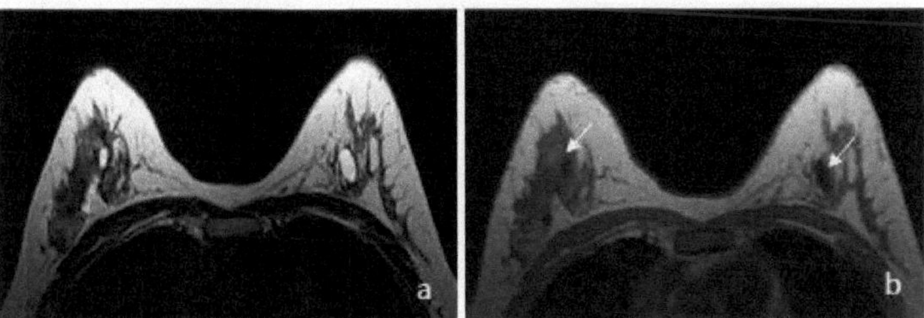

Fig. 121. T2 hypersignal lesion. T2-weighted sequence (a), T1-weighted sequence (b). Multiple oval lesions with circumscribed contours, hypersignal T2, hyposignal T1 (arrows). Histology: Simple cysts

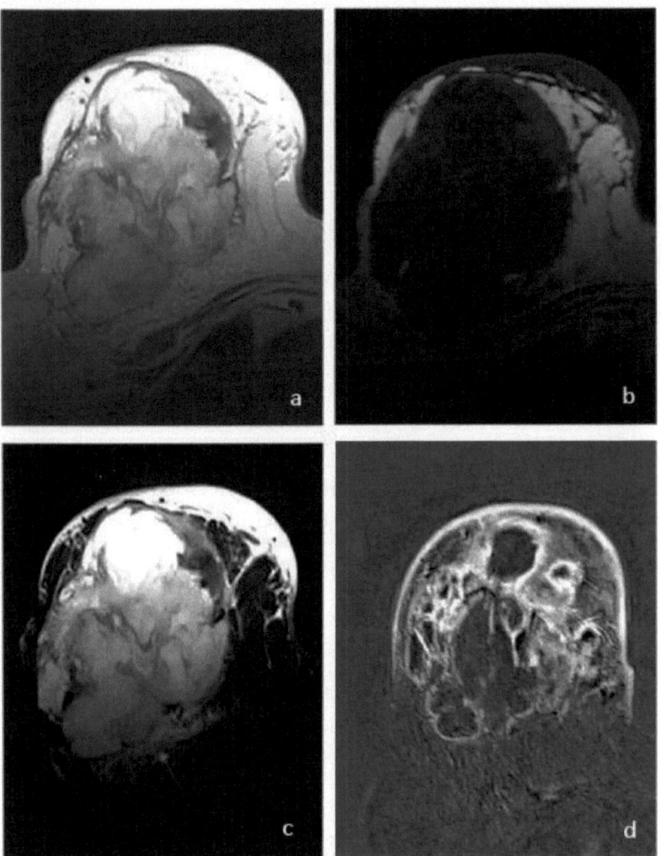

Fig. 122. Low T2 mass. T2-weighted sequence (a), T1-weighted sequence (b), T2 Fat Sat sequence (c) and injected subtraction sequence (d). Voluminous mass of irregular shape and contours, heterogeneous T2 hypersignal, heterogeneous T1 hyposignal, annular enhancement on injected sequences surrounded by peri-lesional oedema in T2 Fat Sat hypersignal (red arrow). Histology: infiltrating lobular carcinoma.

- T1 hypersignal lesion

The T1 signal intensity of the breast lesion is greater than the signal intensity of the breast parenchyma (fig. 123). The T1 hypersignal of a lesion is in favour of benignity. It may be a cytosteatonecrosis lesion or a haemorrhagic cyst (fig. 124). In malignant lesions, liposarcoma presents with a T1 hypersignal due to its fatty component [93, 94].

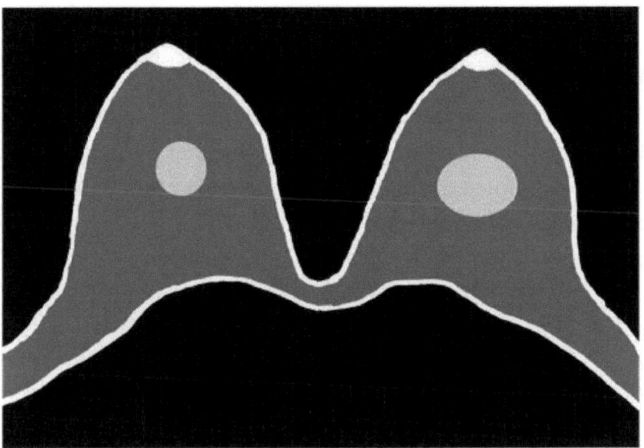

Fig. 123. T1 hypersignal lesion, diagram.

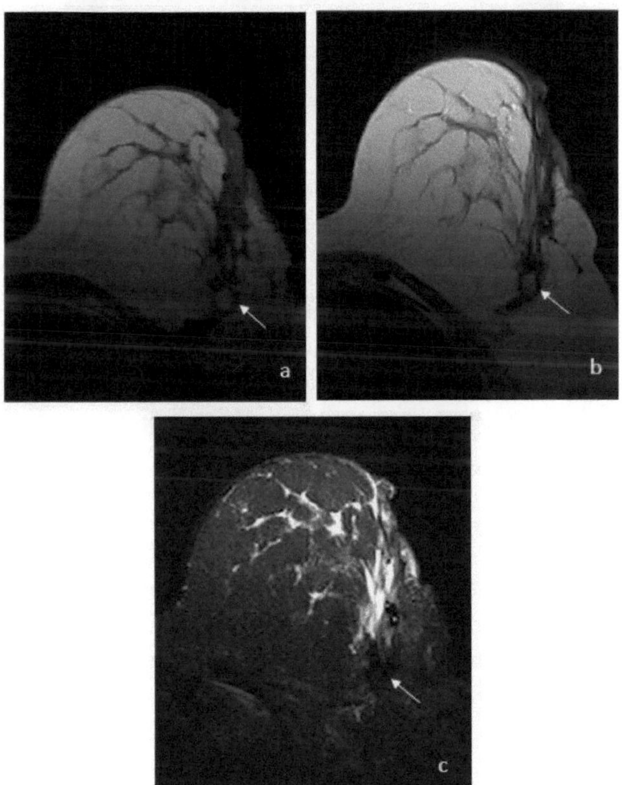

Fig. 124. T1 hypersignal lesion. T2-weighted sequence (a), T1-weighted sequence (b) and T2 Fat Sat-weighted sequence (c). Round lesion with circumscribed contours, T1 and T2 hypersignal and T2 Fat Sat hyposignal,

(arrows). Histology: cytosteatonecrosis.

- # T1 intracanal hypersignal

High signal intensity on intracanal T1-weighted images, unenhanced after injection of contrast medium (fig. 125). This intracanal T1 hypersignal is often associated with a papilloma obstructing the duct or in cases of lactation. A unilateral intracanal high signal may be found following surgery or radiotherapy [81, 82] (fig. 126).

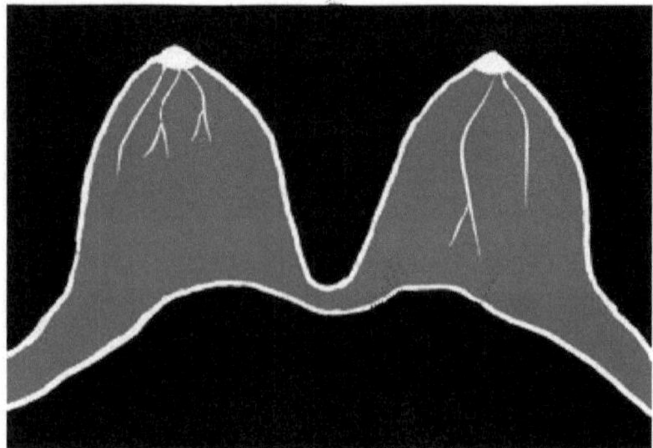

Fig. 125. Intracanal T1 hypersignal, diagram.

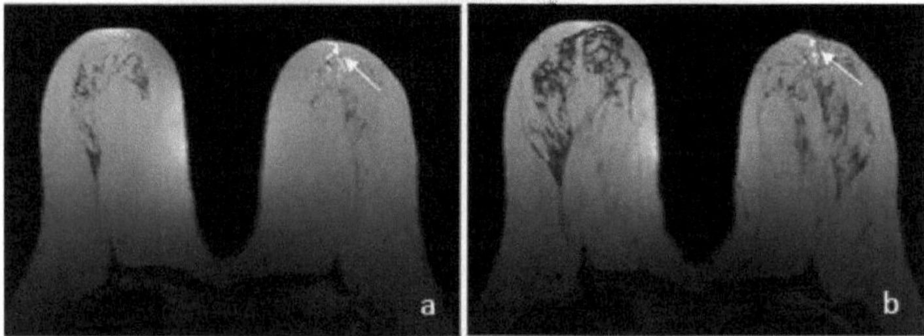

Fig. 126. Intracanal T1 hypersignal. T1-weighted sequence (a+b). Postoperative intra-ductal hypersignal (arrows).

- # Liquid-liquid level

Two levels of intra-lesional fluid (fig. 127). The contents of the lesion may be blood-water, fat-water or water-water with a different protein component. The liquid-liquid level is found in inflammatory cysts, cysts following biopsy or the use of anticoagulants (fig. 128).

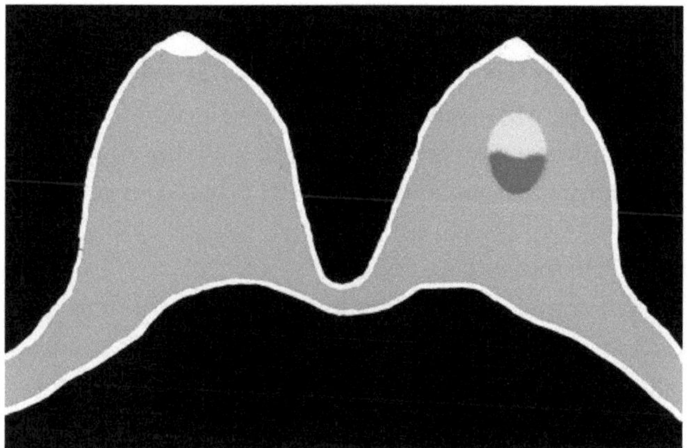

Fig. 127. Liquid-liquid level, diagram.

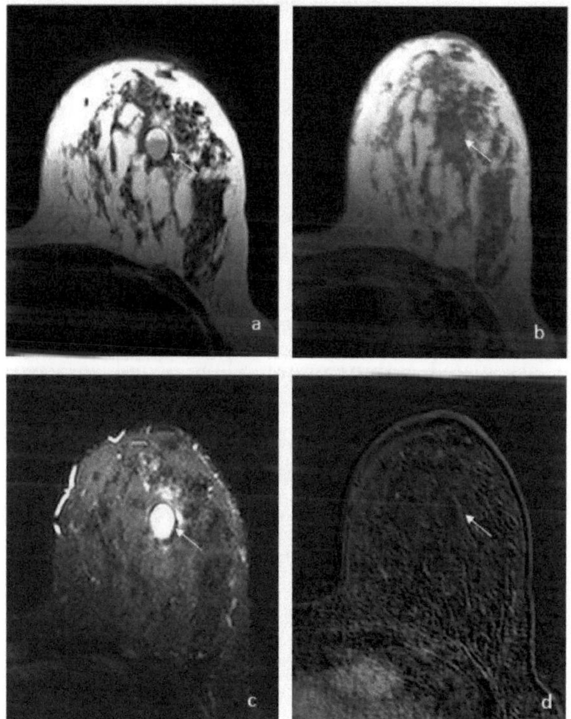

Fig. 128. Liquid-liquid level. T2-weighted sequence (a), T1-weighted sequence (b), T2 Fat Sat sequence (c) and injected subtraction sequence (d). Oval-shaped cystic lesion with circumscribed contours, showing a liquid-liquid level with different signals on T2 and T1 sequences, not enhanced on injected sequences (arrows). Histology: Inflammatory cyst.

6. How to deal with a lesion on breast MRI

Gathering together the MRI signs described above makes it possible to propose a BI-RADS classification of lesions according to the algorithms illustrated below [95]. Diagnostic reasoning in breast MRI is based on determining the type of lesion.

BI-RADS 1 and 2: investigations stopped.

BI-RADS 3: monitoring at 4-6 months by MRI depending on the context (patient at risk) for 2 years unless a mammographic or ultrasound correlation is possible a posteriori (enlarged or centred mammographic images, second-look ultrasound), in order to identify a target lesion for possible sampling guided by these techniques.

BI-RADS 4 and 5: percutaneous sampling should be considered using the technique that allows the abnormality to be seen, such as looking for microcalcifications on mammography in the event of non-mass enhancement, or second-look ultrasound [11]. If there is no correlation with mammography or ultrasound, MRI-guided sampling should be considered.

And of course, a negative MRI does not rule out further investigations, especially in the case of a clinically suspicious lesion or a lesion classified as BI-RADS 4 or 5 on mammography and ultrasound.

6.1. Focus

The management of foci depends on whether they are multiple or single, bilateral or not, associated with pejorative signs or not, in a woman at risk or not. Bilateral and multiple foci in a non-at-risk, non-menopausal woman, with no associated pejorative signs, are in favour of benignity, classified as BI-RADS 2 (fig. 129). Their degree of suspicion increases in women at risk, with a single or few foci or in the case of an adjacent suspicious lesion, the lesion classified as BIRADS 3.

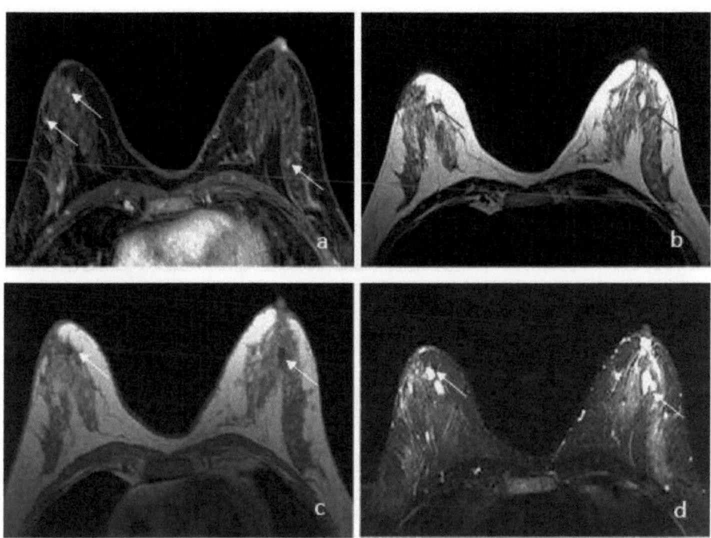

Fig. 129. Multiple foci. Injected sequence (a), T2-weighted sequence (b), T1-weighted sequence (c) and T2 Fat Sat sequence (d). Multiple foci usually due to benign pathology such as areas of fibrocystic mastopathy. Always look for T2 hypersignals (microcyst) (arrows).

6.2. Mass

All the MRI signs of a mass can be used to propose a BIRADS classification according to an algorithm proposed by Chopier et al [95].

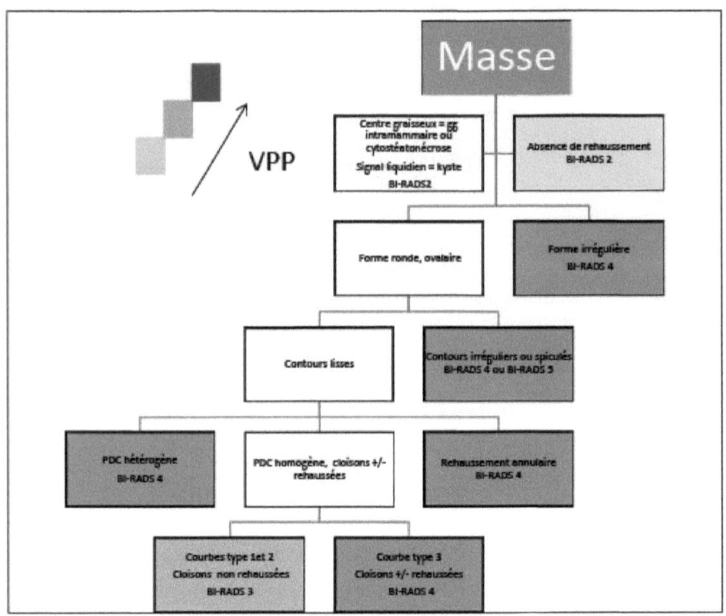

Analysis of the signal on T1 and T2 weighted series helps to gather arguments in favour of benignity and avoids misinterpretation, as in the case of an intramammary lymph node or cytosteatonecrosis lesion, which generally present a fatty centre in T1 hypersignal (figs 130, 131). The absence of enhancement is an argument in favour of benignity classified as BI-RADS 2 (fig. 132).
The irregular shape has the highest inter-observer agreement in favour of malignancy and the oval and round shape in favour of benignity [96] (fig. 133). Contour analysis is the most discriminating feature (fig.134). It is also the most feared inter-observer [97]. The spiculated nature of a mass must therefore be assessed in BI-RADS 5 as in mammography (fig. 135). Ring enhancement is highly suggestive of malignancy, provided that inflammatory cysts (T2 hypersignal), cystadenonecrosis (context and T1 hypersignal) and intra mammary lymph nodes (T1 hypersignal) have been ruled out (fig. 136).

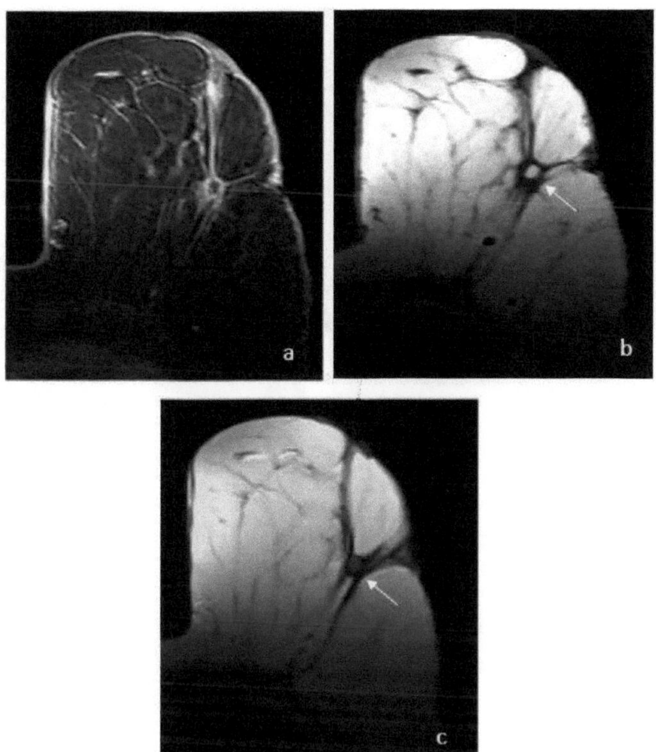

Fig. 130. Injected subtraction sequence (a), T2-weighted sequence (b) and T1-weighted sequence (c). Irregularly shaped lesion with spiculated contours and annular enhancement, classified as BI-RADS 5 on the injected sequences. It is essential to analyse the non-injected T2 and T1 sequences. The lesion is T1, T2 hypersignal (arrows), reclassified as BI-RADS 2. Histology: Cytosteatonecrosis.

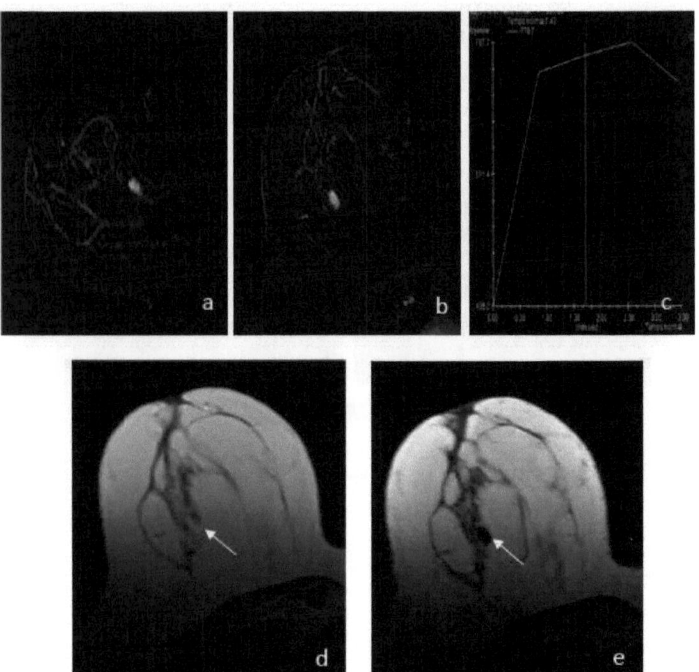

Fig. 131. Injected subtraction sequence (a+b), enhancement curve (c), T2-weighted sequence (d) and T1-weighted sequence (e). Oval-shaped mass with circumscribed contours, homogeneous internal enhancement with type 3 enhancement curve, classified as BI-RADS 4 on the injected sequences. Always look at the non-injected T2 and T1 sequences. Oval mass with a notch, T2 hypersignal, central T1 hypersignal (arrows), reclassified as BI-RADS 2. Histology: Intramammary ganglion.

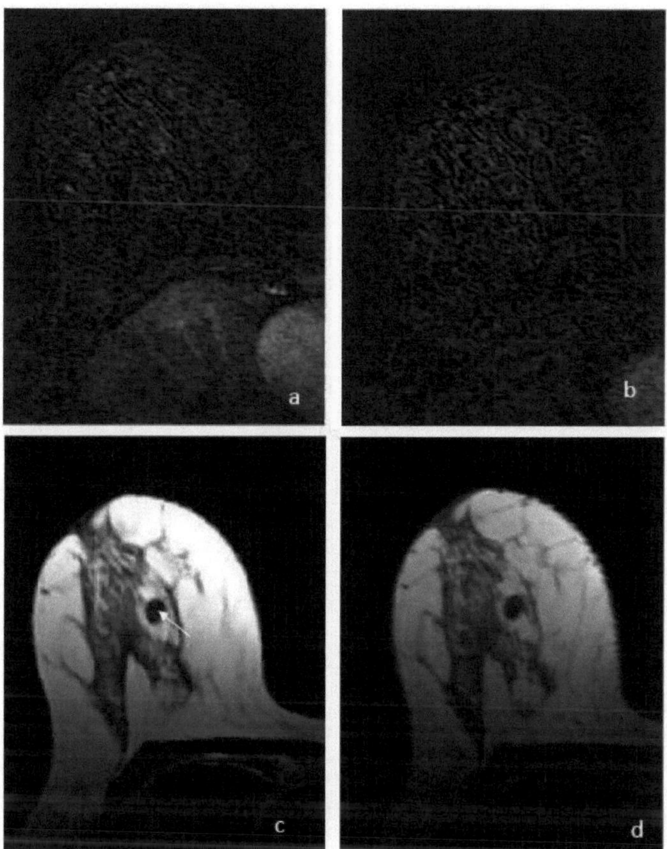

Fig. 132. Injected subtraction sequence (a+b), T2-weighted sequence (c) and T1-weighted sequence (d). Unenhanced mass on non-injected sequences, oval mass, T1 and T2 hyposignal with internal partitions particularly visible in T2 weighting, classified as BI-RADS 2 (arrow). Histology: Fibroadenoma.

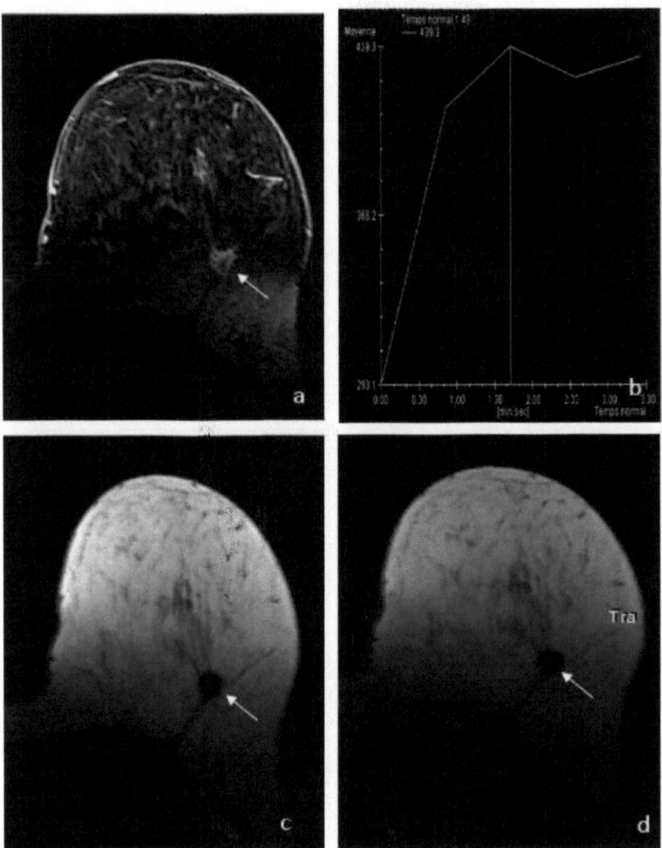

Fig. 133. Injected subtraction sequence (a), enhancement curve (b), T2-weighted sequence (c) and T1-weighted sequence (d). A round, spiculated mass with heterogeneous enhancement on the injected sequences with a type 3 enhancement curve, in T1 and T2 hyposignal, classified as BI-RADS 5 (arrows). Histology: non-specific infiltrating carcinoma.

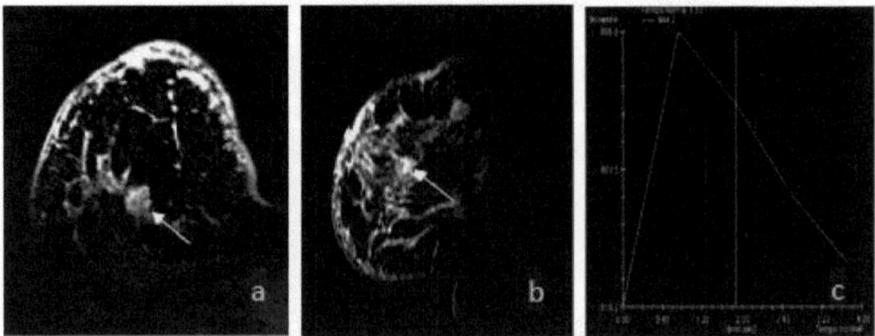

Fig. 134. Injected subtraction sequence, axial section (a), sagittal section (b), enhancement curve (c). Irregularly shaped mass with irregular contours and

heterogeneous enhancement on the injected sequences with a type 3 enhancement curve, classified as BI-RADS 5 (arrows). Histology: non-specific infiltrating carcinoma.

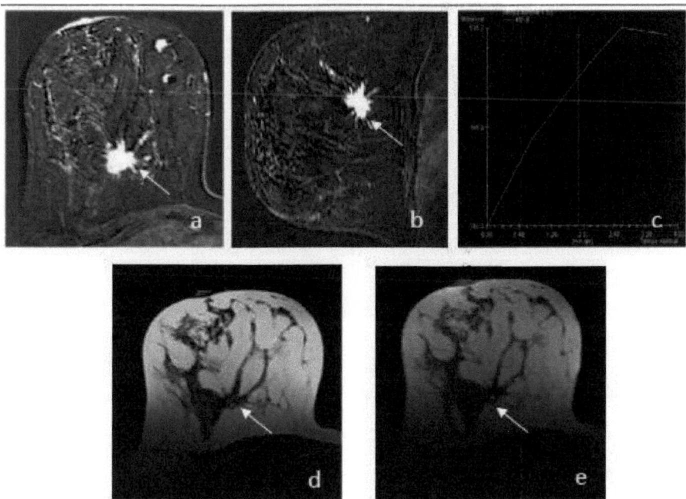

Fig. 135. Subtracted injected sequences, axial section (a), sagittal section (b), enhancement curve (c), T2-weighted sequence (d) and T1-weighted sequence (e). Irregularly shaped mass with spiculated contours and heterogeneous enhancement on the injected sequences with a type 1 enhancement curve, T1 and T2 hyposignal, classified as BI-RADS 5 (arrows). A spiculated mass is classified as BI-RADS 5.
Kinetic analysis is unnecessary.

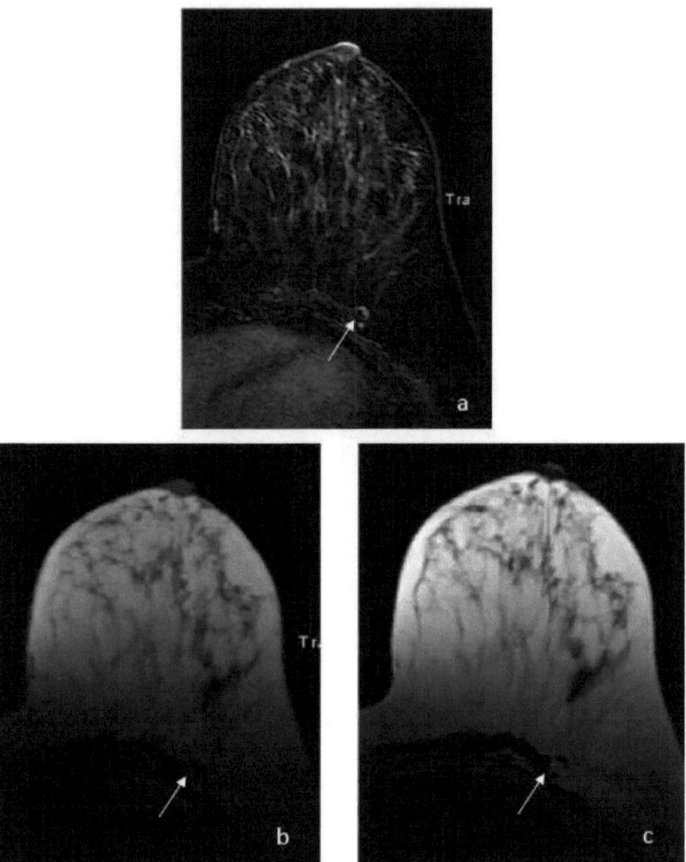

Fig. 136. Injected subtraction sequence (a), T2-weighted sequence (b) and T1-weighted sequence (c). Annular enhancement on the injected sequences. It is important to look at the T2 and T1 sequences, as an oval mass presents with a notch, in T2 hypersignal, central T1 hypersignal (arrows), reclassified as BI-RADS 2. Histology: Intramammary ganglion.

6.3. Raising without mass

All the MRI signs of non-mass enhancement are used to propose a BI-RADS classification according to an algorithm proposed by Chopier et al [95].

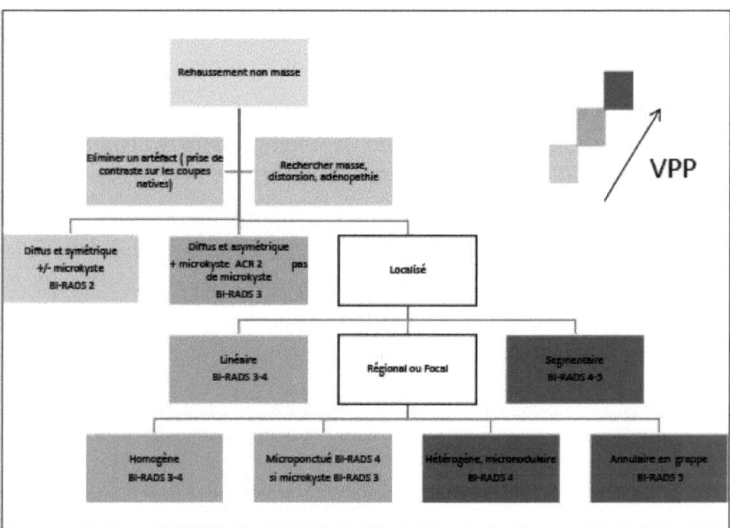

Non-mass enhancement is a process that does not occupy a volume and is not visible on non-injected sequences. It is detected on post-injection sequences.

Before interpretation, always check the patient's hormonal status by questioning (DDR, hormonal treatment) and if necessary repeat the MRI at a different time of the cycle (7th to 14th day of the cycle) or after 2 months of stopping hormonal treatment [98].

It is systematically confirmed that this is not a displacement artefact by visualising this enhancement on the native injected sequences and that no mass is visualised on the non-injected sequences in order to confirm the diagnosis of non-mass enhancement [99].

Non-mass enhancement associated with a suspicious mass or adenopathy is suggestive of malignancy (fig. 137). The presence of microcysts on T2-weighted sequences within a bilateral and symmetrical micropunctate non-mass enhancement is suggestive of fibrocystic mastopathy, classified as BI-RADS 2.

Linear non-mass enhancement is of variable prevalence. The positive predictive value of malignancy varies from 26% to 84% [72]. Linear non-mass enhancement converging towards the micronodular nipple is more suspicious of malignancy than homogeneous linear non-mass enhancement (35% versus 14% of malignancy) [72].

Segmental non-mass enhancement is the most suspicious of the non-mass

enhancements. Its positive predictive value is 67-100% [68]. Segmental non-mass enhancement is classified as BI-RADS 5, as for mammographic microcalcifications. Kinetic analysis is unnecessary.
Regional or focal non-mass enhancement has a positive predictive value of approximately 21% [70]. When the non-mass enhancement is homogeneous or micropunctate, the positive predictive value in favour of malignancy is low, with values of less than 5% when it is homogeneous and 25% when it is micropunctate, but this positive predictive value falls when microcysts are present in T2, suggesting fibrocystic dystrophy [70].
Non-mass enhancement of a heterogeneous, micronodular or annular type is more presumptive of malignancy [70].

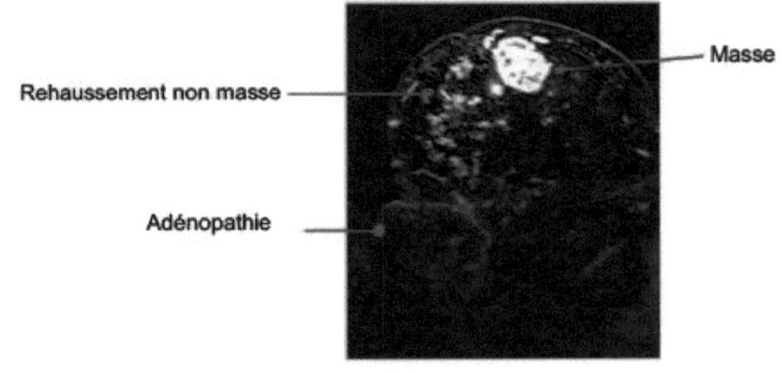

Raising without mass
Adenopathy
Mass

Fig. 137. Injected subtraction sequence. Non-micronodular enhancement associated with a suspicious mass and axillary adenopathy, classified BI-RADS 5.

7. Breast implants

Breast implants are fitted either for reconstructive purposes after mastectomy or for aesthetic purposes such as breast augmentation [100, 101].

7.1. Seat of the breast prosthesis

Two anatomical positions are possible for the breast implant (fig. 138):

- a retroglandular topography, with the implant located behind the fibroglandular tissue and in front of the pectoralis major muscle;
- a retropectoral topography, with the implant located behind the pectoralis major muscle and in front of the pectoralis minor muscle. In cases of breast reconstruction, the implant is placed retropectorally to avoid direct contact of the breast prosthesis with the skin.

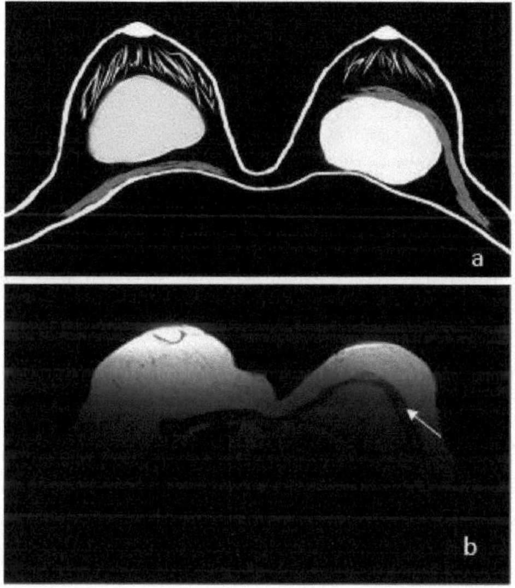

Fig. 138. Seat of the breast prosthesis. Diagram (a), retroglandular topography on the left of the image and retropectoral topography on the right of the image. T2-weighted sequence (b), prosthesis in retropectoral position (arrow).

7.2. Types of breast implants

There are several types of implant. All breast implants are made of an outer shell of "elastomeric" silicone, because of its smooth, textured surface.

7.2.1. Single-compartment breast implants

Two types of implants (fig. 139):

- the breast implants are completely filled with sterile physiological serum (saline solution);

o breast implants are completely filled with cohesive silicone gel. They can have different levels of firmness and provide a texture close to that of a normal breast.

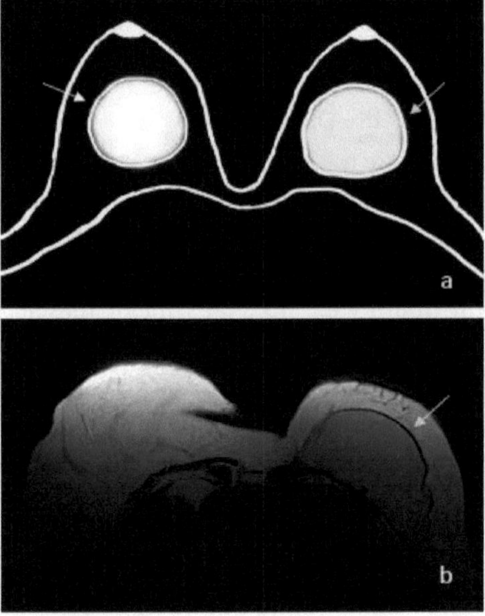

Fig. 139. Single-compartment breast implants. Diagram (a), prosthesis saline solution (white arrow) and silicone prosthesis (yellow arrow). T2-weighted image (b), silicone prosthesis (arrow).

7.2.2. Bicompartmental breast implants

Breast implants, known as Beker prostheses, are made up of a peripheral compartment filled with silicone and a central compartment filled with an inflatable saline solution (fig. 140). This type of prosthesis is generally proposed during breast reconstruction in patients who have a post-therapeutic reduction in skin elasticity or a prosthetic pocket of reduced volume. The central compartment is progressively filled with saline solution until the desired final volume is obtained.

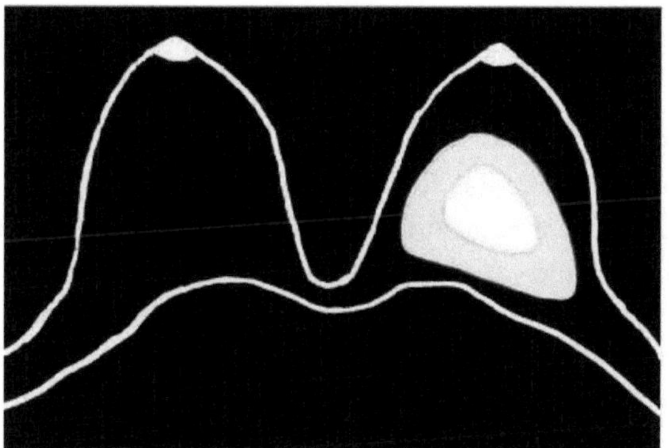

Fig. 140. bicompartmental breast implants, diagram.

7.3. Normal MRI appearance of breast implants

The various MRI sequences (T1 sequences ± injection of gadolinium chelate, TSE T2, STIR and TSE T2 with selective suppression of silicon) make it possible to assess the type of component filling the prosthesis and the type of intra- and extra-prosthetic anomalies.

7.3.1. MRI signals from different prostheses

The saline is in frank hyposignal on the T1-weighted sequence and on the STIR sequence, and in homogeneous hypersignal on the TSE T2 sequence.

The silicone gel shows an intermediate signal on T1- and T2-weighted sequences and a clear hypersignal on the STIR sequence (fig. 141).

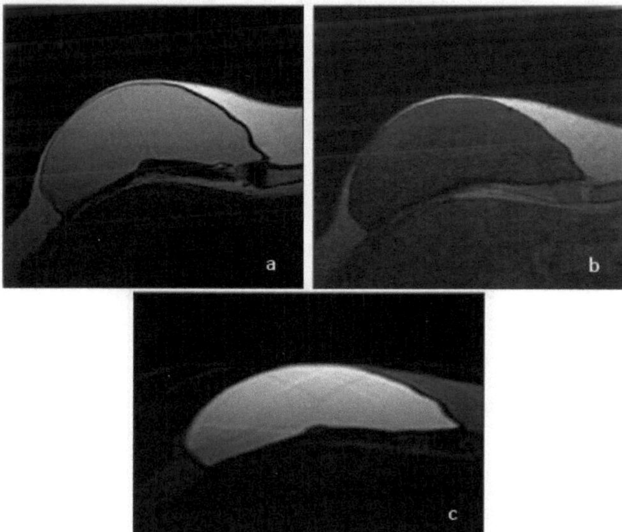

Fig. 141. MRI signal from a silicone prosthesis. T2-weighted sequence (a), T1-

weighted sequence (b) and STIR sequence (c). Intermediate T2 and T1 signal, in frank hypersignal on the STIR sequence.

7.3.2. Radial folds

The presence of normal radial folds in the prosthesis depends on the type of implant, the size, position and thickness of the wall and the degree of capsular retraction [102]. The folds are usually short perpendicular to the wall, generally "simple" and few in number, sometimes "complex", longer and multidirectional (fig. 142). On the STIR sequence, the folds appear as thick black lines extending from the periphery of the prosthesis into the intraprosthetic silicone; this is the main cause of misdiagnosis of intracapsular rupture (Fig. 143).

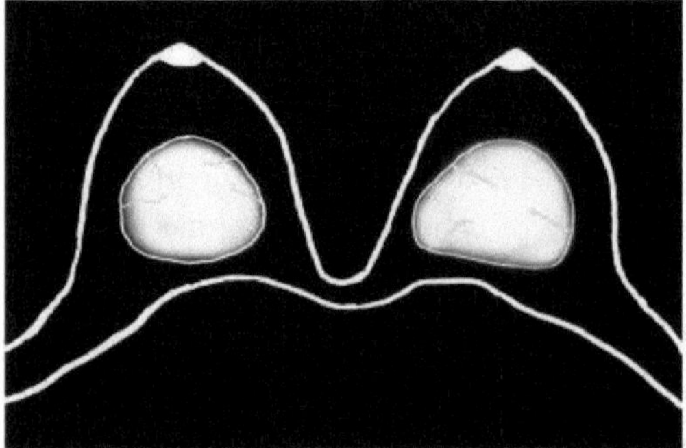

Fig. 142. Radial folds, diagram.

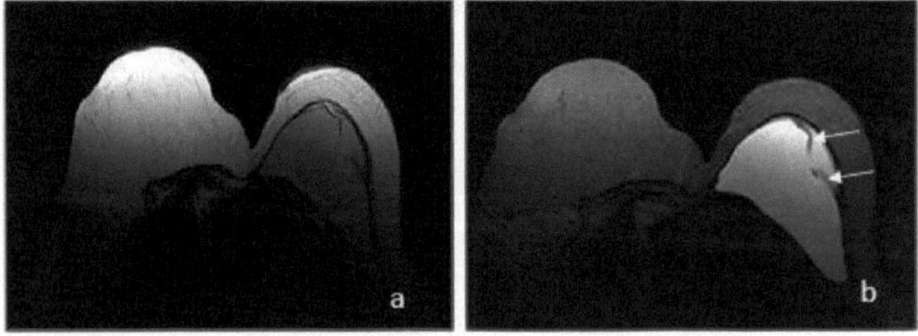

Fig. 143. Radial folds. T2-weighted sequence (a) and STIR sequence (b). Thick, black lines extending from the periphery of the prosthesis into the intraprosthetic silicone (arrows).

7.3.3. Peri-prosthetic effusion

The presence of a periprosthetic reaction effusion is frequent and physiological if small (Fig. 144). It is clearly hyposignal on T1-weighted and STIR sequences and clearly hypersignal on the TSE T2 sequence (Fig. 145). Periprosthetic effusion is frequently found adjacent to folds.

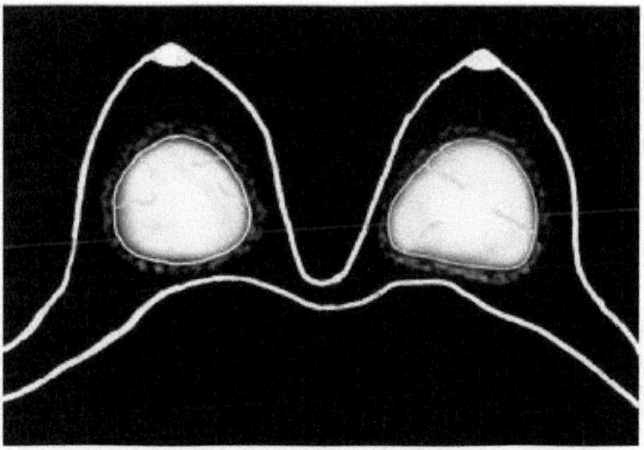

Fig. 144. Peri-prosthetic effusion, diagram.

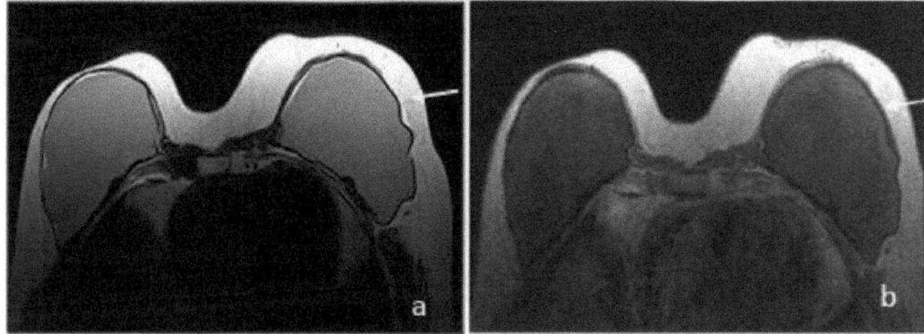

Fig. 145. Periprosthetic effusion. T2-weighted sequence (a) and T1-weighted sequence (b). It is clearly hypersignificant on TSE T2 and clearly hyposignificant on T1-weighted sequences (arrows).

7.4. complications of breast implants

7.4.1. Break

The risk of rupture increases with the age of the prosthesis, but remains rare, varying between 0.01 and 0.3% [103-105]. The average time to rupture is 7.6 years [104]. There are two types of rupture: intra capsular rupture accounts for 80-90% of cases and extra capsular rupture for 10-20% [100].

7.4.1.1. Intracapsular rupture

The rupture may be completely collapsed, partial or minimal, or uncollapsed (Fig. 146).

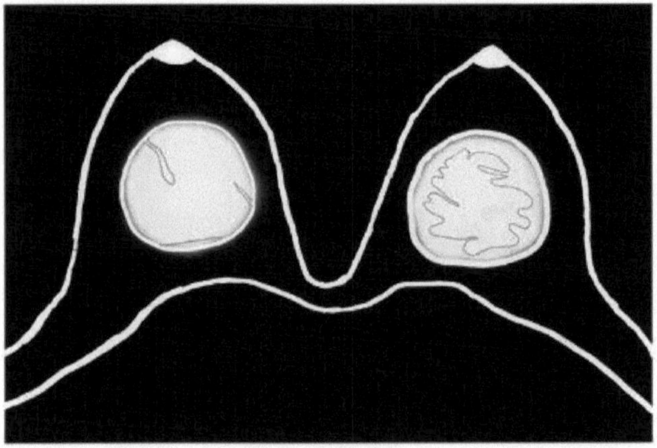

Fig. 146. Intracapsular ruptures with different degrees of envelope collapse, diagram.

Linguine sign

The direct sign of intracapsular rupture, the elastomer completely detached in the silicone gel in the form of multiple multidirectional curvilinear lines in hyposignal T1, T2 and STIR, present clearly defined ends, floating inside the implant [106] (fig. 147). This sign poses a problem of differential diagnosis with complex radial folds, hence the interest of multiplanar analysis.

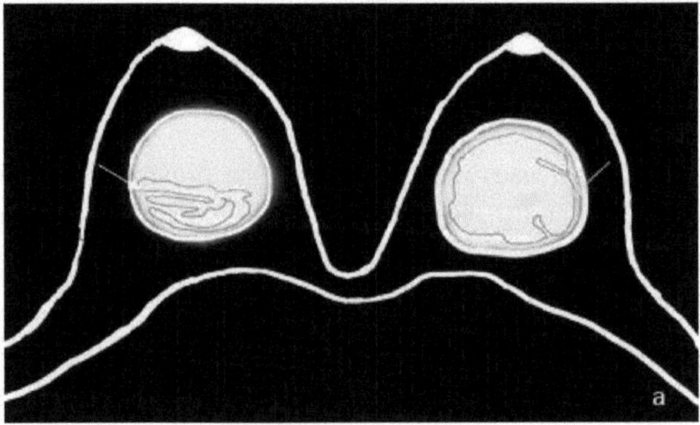

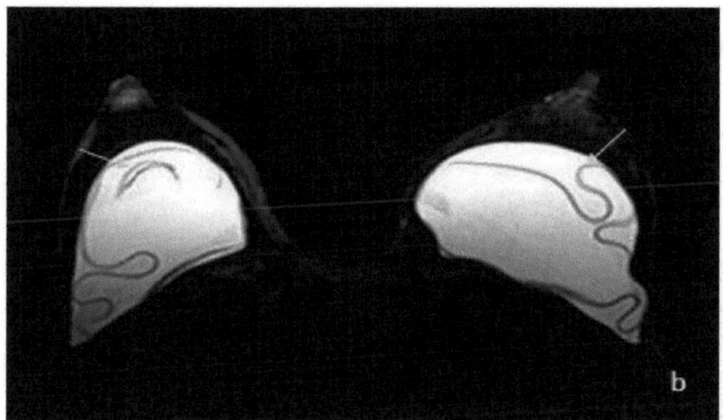

Fig. 147. Linguine sign. Diagram (a), complete collapse (white arrow) and partial collapse (yellow arrow). STIR sequence (b), multidirectional curvilinear lines in STIR hyposignal (arrows).

Subcapsular line sign

Sign of incipient intracapsular rupture. Corresponds to focal detachment of the envelope. T2-hyposignal lines parallel to the edge of the capsule. The ends of the detachment are continuous with the surface of the implant [107] (figs. 148 and 149). Again, this should not be confused with radial folds.

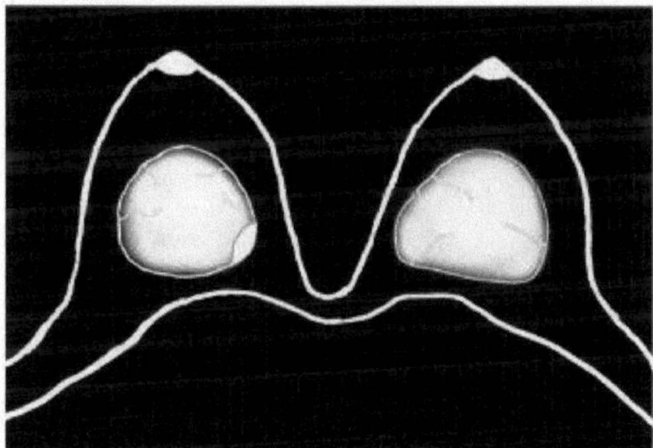

Fig. 148. subcapsular line sign, diagram.

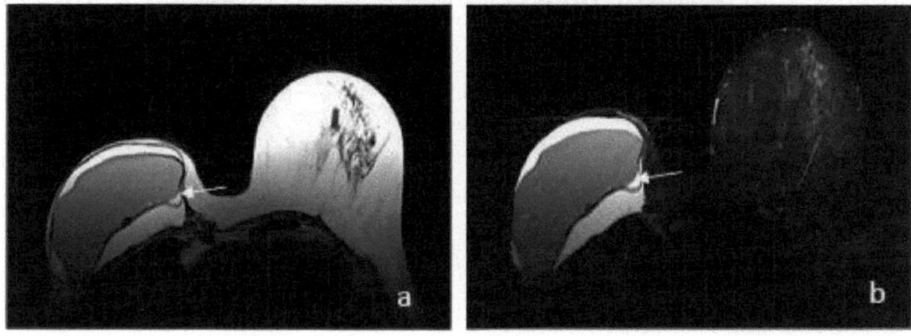

Fig. 149. Subcapsular line sign. T2-weighted sequence (a) and STIR sequence (b). Parallel subcapsular lines in T2 hyposignal and STIR (arrows).

- Keyhole sign or Teardrop sign

Separation of the implant's internal membrane, creating a radial fold that resembles a keyhole [108, 109] (fig. 150).

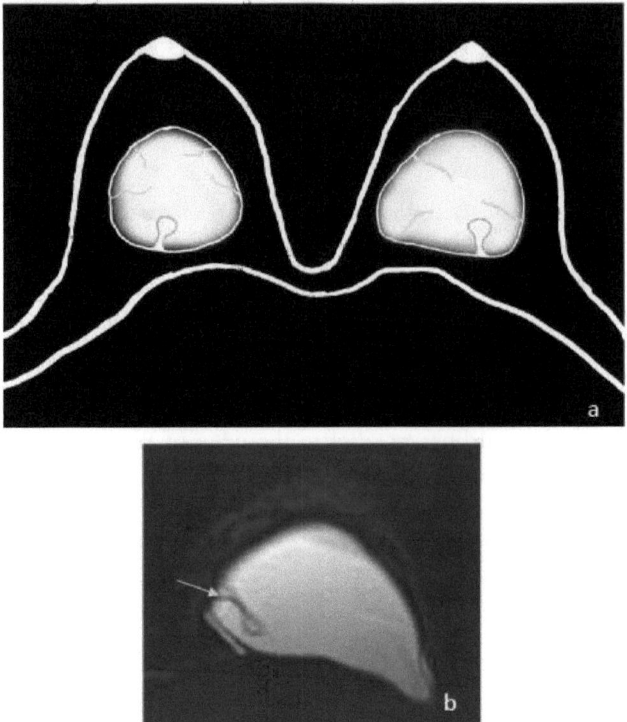

Fig. 150. Keyhole sign. Diagram (a). STIR sequence (b).

Salad oil sign or droplet sign

Signal anomalies within the silicone (fig. 151). This sign can be seen when intra-prosthetic saline is injected intra-operatively to obtain the desired volume, or following steroid treatment in the case of capsular contracture [110, 111].

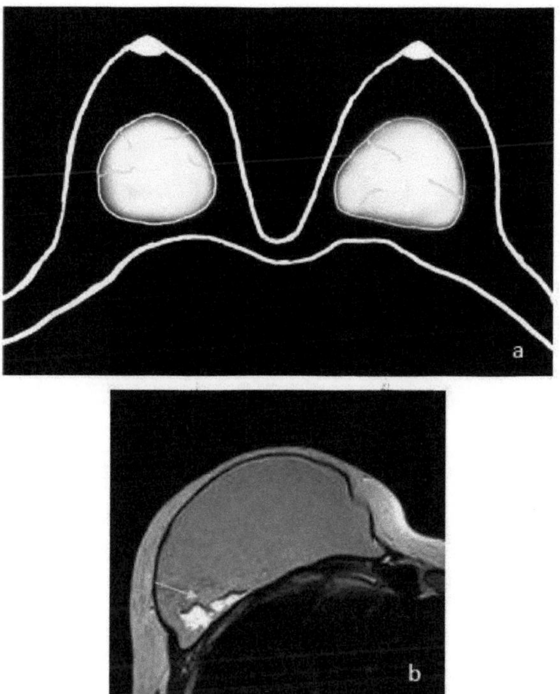

Fig. 151. Salad oil sign. Diagram (a). Sequence in T2 weighting (b). intraprosthetic T2 hypersignals.

7.4.1.2. Extra capsular rupture

Extra capsular rupture is defined by the presence of silicone outside the implant (fig. 152). It is easily detected on the hypersignal STIR sequence, as the suppression of the water signal in this sequence offers the best contrast between the breast parenchyma and the silicone. The siliconoma is the free silicone nodule [112, 113] (fig. 153). It is generally periprosthetic or continuous with the prosthesis, but may migrate to the axillary lymph nodes or the chest wall.

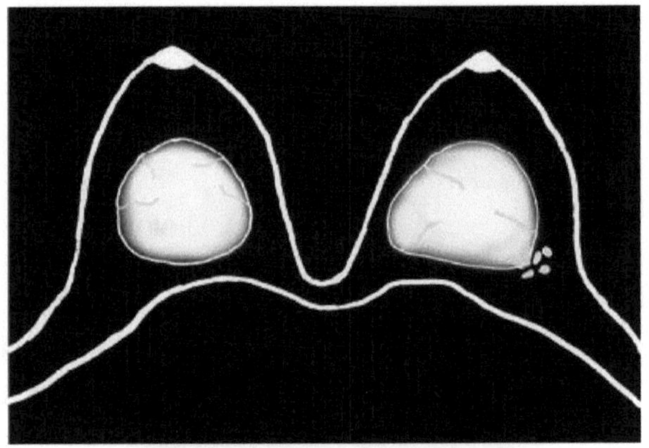

Fig. 152. Extracapsular rupture, diagram.

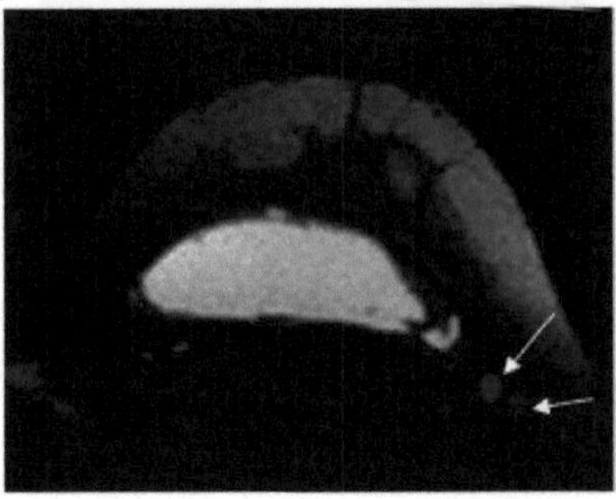

Fig. 153. Siliconoma STIR sequence. Hypersignal nodule (arrows).

7.4.2. Periprosthetic tumour recurrence

The risk of recurrence is due to incomplete resection of breast tissue during mastectomy [114, 115]. On MRI, it presents as a mass in hyposignal on T1 and T2 sequences, enhanced after injection of contrast product and associated with a large periprosthetic effusion (fig. 154).

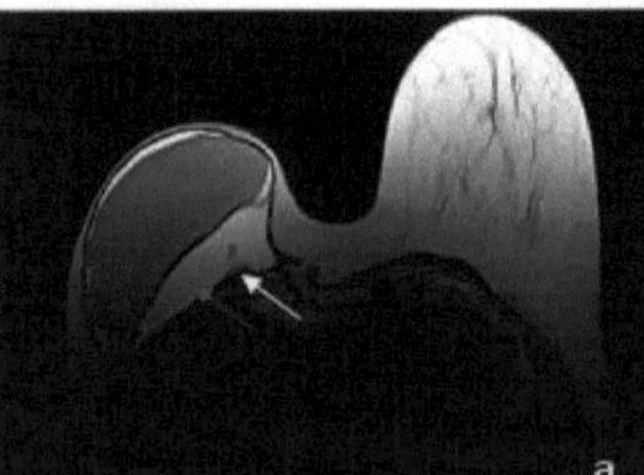

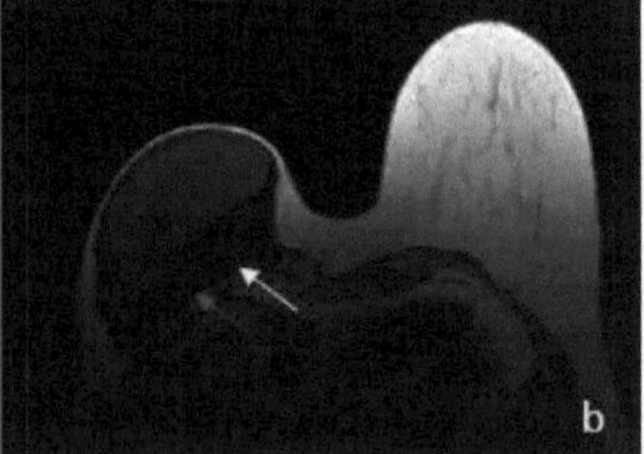

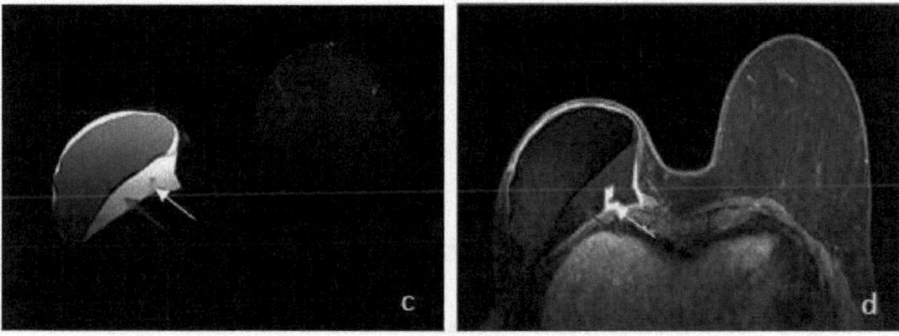

Fig. 154. Periprosthetic tumour recurrence. T2-weighted sequence (a), T2-weighted sequence (b).
T1-weighted sequence (b), T2 Fat Sat sequence (c) and injected subtraction sequence (d). Irregular mass in T1 and T2 hypopositivity, with heterogeneous enhancement on the injected sequences (white arrows). Significant periprosthetic effusion (red arrows).

Reference

1. Levy L, Michelin J, Teman G, Martin B, Dana A, Lacan A, Meyer D. Techniques d'exploration radiologique du sein (mammographie, échographie, IRM). Encycl Méd Chir 2001; 34-800-A-10.
2. Banks, E., Reeves, G., Beral, V., Bull, D., Crossley, B., Simmonds, M., . . Patnick, J. Influence of personal characteristics of individual women on sensitivity and specificity of mammography in the Million Women Study: Cohort study. BMJ, 2004; 329, 477-482.
3. Heywang-Kobrunner S H, Schreer I, Bassler R, Perlet C, Viehweg P. Mammography. Imagerie diagnostique du sein : Mammographie, échographie, IRM, techniques interventionnelles 2007 ; 19-97.
4. Barry DA, Cronin KA, Plevritis SK, Fryback DG,Clarke L, Zelen M, et al. Effect of screening and adjuvant therapy on mortality from breast cancer. N Emgl J Med. 2005;353 (17): 1784-92.
5. Tabar L, Yen MF, Vitak B, Chen H-HT, Smith RA, Duffy SW. Mammography service screening and martality in breast cancer patients: 20-year follow-up before and after introduction of screening. lANCET. 2003; 361 (9367) : 1405-10.
6. Hellquist BN, Duffy SW, Abdsaleh S, Bjorneld L, Bordas P, Tabar L, et al. Effectiveness of population-based service screening with mammography forwomen ages 40 to 49 years evaluation of the Swedish Mammography in Young Women (SCRY) cohort. Cancer. 2011; 117 (4) : 714-22.
7. Kerlikowske K, Grady D, Barclay J, Sickles EA, Ernster V. Effect of age, breast density, and Family history on the sensitivity of first screening mammography. JAMA. 1996; 276 (1) : 33-8.
8. Mandelson M, oestreicher N, Porter PL,White D, Finder CA, Taplin SH, et al. Breast density as a predictor of mammographic detection: comparison of interval and screen detected cancers. J Natl Cancer Inst. 2000; 92 (13): 1081-7.
9. Folkman J. The influence of angiogenesis research on management of patients with breast cancer. Breast Cancer Res Treat 1995;36:109-18.
10. Folkman J. The role of angiogenesis in tumor growth. Semin Cancer Biol 1992;3:65-71.
11. Kuhl C. The current status of breast MR imaging. Part I. Choice of technique, image interpretation, diagnostic accuracy, and transfer to clinical practice. Radiology. 2007 Aug;244(2):356-78.
12. Hillman BJ, Harms SE, Stevens G, Stough RG, Hollingsworth AB, Kozlowski KF, et al. Diagnostic performance of a dedicated 1.5 T breast MR imaging system. Radiology 2012;265:51-8. http://dx.doi.org/10.1148/radiol.12110600.
13. Baur A, Bahrs SD, Speck S, Wietek BM, Krämer B, Vogel U, et al. Breast MRI of pure ductal carcinoma in situ: sensitivity of diagnosis and influence of lesion characteristics. Eur J Radiol 2013;82:1731-7. http://dx.doi.org/10.1016/j.ejrad.2013. 05.002.
14. Hammersleya JA, Partridgeb SC, Blitzera GC, Deitcha S, Rahbarb H. Management of high-risk breast lesions found on mammogram or ultrasound: the value of contrast- enhanced MRI to exclude malignancy. Clinical Imaging 49; 2018; 174-180.
15. Sardanelli F, Boetes C, Borisch B, Decker T, Federico M, Gilbert FJ, et al. Magnetic resonance imaging of the breast: recommendations from the EUSOMA working group. Eur J Cancer. 2010 May;46(8):1296-316.
16. Kriege M, Brekelmans CT, Boetes C, Besnard PE, Zonderland HM, Obdeijn IM, et al. Efficacy of MRI and mammography for breast-cancer screening in women with a familial or genetic predisposition. N Engl J Med 2004;351:427-37.
17. Kuhl CK, Schrading S, Leutner CC et al. Mammography, breast ultrasound, and magnetic resonance imaging for surveillance of women at high familial risk for breast cancer. J Clin Oncol 2005;23:8469-76.
18. Warner E, Plewes DB, Hill KA, et al. Sur- veillance of BRCA1 and BRCA2 Mutation carriers with Magnetic Resonance Imaging, Ultra- sound, Mammographic and clinical examination. JAMA 2004;292:1317-25.
19. Podo F, Sardanelli F, Canese R et al. The Italian multi-centre project on evaluation of MRI and

other imaging modalities in early detection of breast cancer in subjects at high genetic risk. J Exp Clin Cancer Res 2002;21:115-24.
20. Tilanus-Linthorst MM, Bartels CC, Ob- deijn AI et al. Earlier detection of breast cancer by surveillance of women at familial risk. Eur J Cancer 2000;36:514-19.
21. Kriege M, Brekelmans CT, Boetes C et al. Efficacy of MRI and mammography for breastcancer screening in women with a familial or gene- tic predisposition. N Engl J Med 2004;351:427-37.
22. Leach MO, Boggis CR and Dixon AK et al. Screening with magnetic resonance imaging and mammography of a UK population at high familial risk of breast cancer a prospective multicentre co-hort study (MARIBS). Lancet 2005;365:1769-78.
23. Lehman CD, Blume JD, Weatherall P et al. Screening women at high risk for breast cancer with mammography and magnetic resonance imaging. Cancer 2005;103:1898-1905.
24. Morris EA, Liberman L, Ballon DJ et al. MRI of occult breast carcinoma in a high-risk population. AJR Am J Roentgenol 2003;181: 619-26.
25. Kuhl CK, Kuhl W, Schild H. Management of women at high risk for breast cancer. Breast 2005; 14: 480-486.
26. Hagen AI, Kvistad KA, Maehle L, Holmen MM, Aase H, Styr B, et al. Sensitivity of MRI versus conventional screening in the diagnosis of BRCA-associated breast cancer in a national prospective series. Breast 2007;16:367-74.
27. Sardanelli F, Podo F. Breast MR imaging in women at high-risk of breast cancer. Is something changing in early breast cancer detection? Eur Radiol 2007;17:873-87.
28. Henry-Tillman RS, Harms SE, Westbrook KC, Korourian S, Klimberg VS. Role of breast magnetic resonance imaging in determining breast as a source of unknown metastatic lymphadenopathy. Am J Surg 1999;178:496-500.
29. Olson JA, Morris EA, Van Zee KJ, Linehan DC, Borgen PI. Magnetic resonance imaging facilitates breast conservation for occult breast cancer. Ann Surg Oncol 2000;7:411-5.
30. Lieberman S, Sella T, Maly B, Sosna J, Uziely B, Sklair-Levy M. Breast magnetic resonance imaging characteristics in women with occult primary breast carcinoma. Isr Med Assoc J 2008;10:448-52.
31. KoEY, Han B-K, Shin JH, Kang SS. Breast MRI for evaluating patients with metastatic axillary lymph node and initially negative mammography and sonography. Korean J Radiol 2007;8:382-9.
32. Buchanan CL, Morris EA, Dorn PL, Borgen PI, Van Zee KJ. Utility of breast magnetic resonance imaging in patients with occult primary breast cancer. Ann Surg Oncol 2005;12:1045-53.
33. Sardanelli F, Giuseppetti GM, Panizza P, Bazzocchi M, Fausto A, Simonetti G, et al. Sensitivity of MRI versus mammography for detecting foci of multifocal, multicentric breast cancer in Fatty and dense breasts using the whole-breast pathologic examination as a gold standard. AJR Am J Roentgenol 2004;183:1149-57.
34. Sardanelli F, Bacigalupo L, Carbonaro L, Esseridou A, Giuseppetti GM, Panizza P, et al. What is the sensitivity of mammography and dynamic MR imaging for DCIS if the wholebreast histopathology is used as a reference standard? Radiol Med 2008;113:439-51.
35. Turnbull L, Brown S, Harvey I, Olivier C, Drew P, Napp V, et al. Comparative effectiveness of MRI in breast cancer (COMICE) trial: a randomised controlled trial. Lancet 2010;375:563-71.
36. Peters NHGM, vanEsser S, van den BoschMa. a. J, Storm RK, Plaisier PW, van Dalen T, et al. Preoperative MRI and surgical management in patients with nonpalpable breast cancer: the MONET - randomized controlled trial. Eur J Cancer 2011;47:879-86.
37. Straver ME, van Adrichem JC, Rutgers EJ, Rodenhuis S, Linn SC, Loo CE, et al. Neoadjuvant systemic therapy in patients with operable primary breast cancer: more benefits than breast-conserving therapy. Ned Tijdschr Geneeskd 2008;152:2519-25.
38. Londero V, Bazzocchi M, Del Frate C, Puglisi F, Di Loreto C, Francescutti G, et al. Locally advanced breast cancer: comparison of mammography, sonography and MR imaging in evaluation of residual disease in women receiving neoadjuvant chemotherapy. Eur Radiol 2004;14:1371-9.

39. Yeh E, Slanetz P, Kopans DB, Rafferty E, Georgian-Smith D, Moy L, et al. Prospective comparison of mammography, sonography, and MRI in patients undergoing neoadjuvant chemotherapy for palpable breast cancer. AJR Am J Roentgenol 2005;184:868-77.

40. Wasser K, Klein SK, Fink C, Junkermann H, Sinn HP, Zuna I, et al. Evaluation of neoadjuvant chemotherapeutic response of breast cancer using dynamic MRI with high temporal resolution. Eur Radiol 2003;13:80-7.

41. Bhattacharyya M, Ryan D, Carpenter R, Vinnicombe S, Gallagher CJ. Using MRI to plan breast-conserving surgery following neoadjuvant chemotherapy for early breast cancer. Br J Cancer 2008;98:289-93.

42. Akazawa K, Tamaki Y, Taguchi T, Tanji Y, Miyoshi Y, Kim SJ, et al. Preoperative evaluation of r esidual tumor extent by three-dimensional magnetic resonance imaging in breast cancer patients treated with neoadjuvant chemotherapy. Breast J 2006;12: 130-7.

43. Pinel-Giroux FM, El Khoury MM, Trop I, Bernier C, David J, Lalonde L. Breast reconstruction: review of surgical methods and spectrum of imaging findings. Radiographics 2013;33:435-53.

44. Margolis NE, Morley C, Lotfi P, Shaylor SD, Palestrant S, Moy L, et al. Update on imaging of the postsurgical breast. Radiographics 2014;34:642-60.

45. Morakkabati N, Leutner CC, Schmiedel A, Schild HH, Kuhl CK. Breast MR imaging during or soon after radiation therapy. Radiology 2003;229:893-901.

46. Belli P, Costantini M, Romani M, Marano P, Pastore G. Magnetic resonance imaging in breast cancer recurrence. Breast Cancer Res Treat 2002;73:223-35.

47. Preda L,Villa G, Rizzo S, Bazzi L, Origgi D, Cassano E, et al. Magnetic resonance mammography in the evaluation of recurrence at the prior lumpectomy site after conservative surgery and radiotherapy. Breast Cancer Res 2006;8:R53.

48. Maxwell GP, Van Natta BW, Murphy DK, Slicton A, Bengtson BP. Natrelle style 410 form-stable silicone breast implants: core study results at 6 years. Aesthetic Surg J 2012;32:709-17.

49. Hammond DC, Migliori MM, Caplin DA, Garcia ME, Phillips CA. Mentor Contour Profile Gel implants: clinical outcomes at 6 years. Plast Reconstr Surg 2012;129:1381-91.

50. Stevens WG, Harrington J, Alizadeh K, Berger L, Broadway D, Hester TR, et al. Five-year follow-up data from the U.S. clinical trial for Sientra's U.S. Food and Drug Administration- approved Silimed® brand round and shaped implants with high-strength silicone gel. Plast Reconstr Surg 2012;130:973-81.

51. Di Benedetto G, Cecchini S, Grassetti L, Baldassarre S, Valeri G, Leva L, et al. Comparative study of breast implant rupture using mammography, sonography, and magnetic resonance imaging: correlation with surgical findings. Breast J 2008;14:532-7.

52. 1. Speirs V, Shaaban AM, et al. The rising incidence of male breast cancer. *Breast Cancer Res Treat.* 2008 May;115(2):429-30.

53. Nguyen C, Kettler MD, Swirsky ME, Miller VI, Scott C, Krause R, et al. Male breast disease: pictorial review with radiologic-pathologic correlation. Radiographics 2013;33:763-79.

54. El Khouli RH, Macura KJ, Kamel IR, Bluemke DA, Jacobs MA. The effects of applying breast compression in dynamic contrast material-enhanced MR imaging. Radiology 2014;272:79-90.

55. Wilkinson J, Appleton CM, Margenthaler JA. Utility of breast MRI for evaluation of residual disease following excisional biopsy. J Surg Res 2011;170:233-9.

56. Lee JM, Orel SG, Czerniecki BJ, Solin LJ, Schnall MD. MRI before reexcision surgery in patients with breast cancer. AJR Am J Roentgenol 2004;182:473-80.

57. Orel SG, Reynolds C, Schnall MD, Solin LJ, Fraker DL, Sullivan DC. Breast carcinoma:MRimaging before re-excisional biopsy. Radiology 1997;205:429-36.

58. Mann RM,Kuhl CK, Kinkel K, Boetes C. Breast MRI: guidelines from the European Society of Breast Imaging. Eur Radiol 2008;18:1307-18.

59. Szumowski J, Coshow W, Li F, Coombs B, Quinn SF. Double-echo three-point-Dixon method

for fat suppression MRI. Magn Reson Med 1995;34(1):120-4.
60. Sharma U, Danishad KK, Seenu V, Jagannathan NR. Longitudinal study of the assessment by MRI and diffusion-weighted imaging of tumor response in patients with locally advanced breast cancer undergoing neoadjuvant chemotherapy. NMR Biomed 2009;22:104-13.
61. Iacconi C, Giannelli M, Marini C, Cilotti A, Moretti M, Viacava P, et al. The role of mean diffusivity (MD) as a predictive index of the response to chemotherapy in locally advanced breast cancer: a preliminary study. Eur Radiol 2010;20:303-8.
62. Negendank W. Studies of human tumors by MRS: a review. NMR Biomed 1992;5(5):303-24.
63. Bartella L, Morris EA, Dershaw DD, Liberman L, Thakur SB, Moskowitz C, et al. Proton MR spectroscopy with choline peak as malignancy marker improves positive predictive value for breast cancer diagnosis: preliminary study. Radiology 2006;239(3):686-92.
64. Baek HM, Chen JH, Nalcioglu O, Su MY. Proton MR spectroscopy for monitoring early treatment response of breast cancer to neo-adjuvant chemotherapy. Ann Oncol 2008;19(5): 1022-4.
65. D'Orsi C.J., Sickles E.A., Mendelson E.B. and Morris E.A. ACR BI-RADS Atlas: Breast Imaging Re-porting and Data System. American College of Radiology Reston, VA, USA; 2013.
66. Garbay JR. Anatomy of the breast and axillary region. Breast Cancer Surgery: Diagnostic, Curative and Reconstructive 1997; 3-17.
67. Gallardo X, Sentis M, Castaner E, et al. Enhancement of intramammary lymph nodes with lymphoid hyperplasia: a potential pitfall in breast MRI. Eur Radiol. 1998;8: 1662-5.
68. Agrawal G, Su MY, Nalcioglu O, Feig SA, Chen JH. Significance of breast lesion descriptors in the ACR BI-RADS MRI lexicon. Cancer 2009 ;115(7):1363-1380.
69. Kuhl CK. Concepts for differential diagnosis in breast MR imaging. Magn Reson Imaging Clin N Am. 2006;14:305-328.
70. Schnall MD, Blume J, Bluemke DA et al. Diagnostic architectural and dynamic features at breast MR imaging: multicenter study. Radiology 2006 ;238(1):42-53.
71. Nunes LW, Schnall MD, Siegelman ES et al. Diagnostic performance characteristics of architectural features revealed by high spatial-resolution MR imaging of the breast. Am J Roentgenol 1997 ;169(2):409-415.
72. Liberman L, Morris EA, Dershaw DD, Abramson AF, Tan LK. Ductal enhancement on MR imaging of the breast. Am J Roentgenol 2003 ;181(2):519-525.
73. Tozaki M, Fukuda K. High-spatial-resolution MRI of non-masslike breast lesions: interpretation model based on BI-RADS MRI descriptors. AJR Am J Roentgenol 2006 ;187(2):330-337.
74. *Stavros T. Breast ultrasound Lippincott and Williams, and Wilkins 2004.*
75. Kuhl CK, Mielcareck P, Klaschik S, Leutner C, Wardelmann E, Gieseke J, Schild HH. Dynamic breast MR imaging: are signal intensity time course data useful for differential diagnosis of enhancing lesions? Radiology. 1999 Apr;211(1):101-10.
76. Dietzel M, Baltzer PA, Vag T, Gajda M, Camara O, Kaiser WA. The hook sign for differential diagnosis of malignant from benign lesions in magnetic resonance mammography: experience in a study of 1084 histologically verified cases. Acta Radiol. 2010.
77. Sequeiros RB, Reinikainen H, Sequeiros AM, et al. MR-guided breast biopsy and hook wire marking using a low-field (0.23 T) scanner with optical instrument tracking. Eur Radiol 2007; 17:813-819.
78. Renz DM, Baltzer PA, Böttcher J, Thaher F, Gajda M, Camara O, Runnebaum IB, Kaiser WA. Inflammatory breast carcinoma in magnetic resonance imaging: a comparison with locally advanced breast cancer. Acad Radiol. 2008 Feb;15(2):209-21.
79. Preda L, Villa G, Rizzo S, et al. Magnetic resonance mammography in the evaluation of recurrence at the prior lumpectomy site after conservative surgery and radiotherapy. Breast Cancer Res 2006; 8:R53.

80. Rieber A, Tomczak RJ, Mergo PJ, Wenzel V, Zeitler H, Brambs HJ. MRI of the breast in the differential diagnosis of mastitis versus inflammatory carcinoma and follow-up. J Comput Assist Tomogr 1997; 21:128-132.
81. Forrai G, Polgar C, Zana K, et al. The role of STIR MRI sequence in the evaluation of the breast following conservative surgery and radiotherapy. Neoplasma 2001; 48:7-11.
82. Preda L, Villa G, Rizzo S, et al. Magnetic resonance mammography in the evaluation of recurrence at the prior lumpectomy site after conservative surgery and radiotherapy. Breast Cancer Res 2006; 8:R53.
83. Shirakawa K, Kobayashi H, Heike Y, et al. Hemodynamics in vasculogenic mimicry and angiogenesis of inflammatory breast cancer xenograft. Cancer Res 2002; 62:560-566.
84. Shirakawa K, Kobayashi H, Sobajima J, Hashimoto D, Shimizu A, Wakasugi H. Inflammatory breast cancer: vasculogenic mimicry and its hemodynamics of an inflammatory breast cancer xenograft model. Breast Cancer Res 2003; 5:136-139.
85. Lee KW, Chung SY, Yang I, et al. Inflammatory breast cancer: imaging findings. Clin Imaging 2005; 29:22-25.
86. Belli P, Costantini M, Romani M, Pastore G. Role of magnetic resonance imaging in inflammatory carcinoma of the breast. Rays 2002; 27:299-305.
87. Chow CK. Imaging in inflammatory breast carcinoma. Breast Dis 2005; 22:45-54.
88. Cervinka V, St'astny K, Havlicek K, Nechvatal L. [An axillary metastasis as the first sign of the breast carcinoma - a case review]. Rozhl Chir 2006; 85:71-73.
89. Graham SJ, Bronskill MJ. MR measurement of relative water content and multicomponent T2 relaxation in human breast. Magn Reson Med 1996; 35:706-715.
90. Graham SJ, Stanchev PL, Bronskill MJ. Criteria for analysis of multicomponent tissue T2 relaxation data. Magn Reson Med 1996; 35:370-378.
91. Kvistad KA, Lundgren S, Fjosne HE, Smenes E, Smethurst HB, Haraldseth O. Differentiating benign and malignant breast lesions with T2*-weighted first pass perfusion imaging. Acta Radiol 1999; 40:45-51.
92. Yuen S, Uematsu T, Kasami M, et al. Breast carcinomas with strong high-signal intensity on T2-weighted MR images: pathological characteristics and differential diagnosis. J Magn Reson Imaging 2007; 25:502-510.
93. Diekmann F, Rudolph B, Winzer KJ, Bick U. Liposarcoma of the breast arising within a phyllodes tumor. J Comput Assist Tomogr 1999; 23:764-766.
94. Mazaki T, Tanak T, Suenaga Y, Tomioka K, Takayama T. Liposarcoma of the breast: a case report and review of the literature. Int Surg 2002; 87:164-170
95. J Chopier, C Lafont, C Salem, N Perrot, C Marsault,IThomassin Naggara. Tips and tricks in breast MRI. Journée française de radiologie 2009.
96. Ikeda DM. Progress report from the American College of Radiology Breast MR Imaging Lexicon Committee. Magn Reson Imaging Clin N Am. 2001 May;9(2):295-302.
97. Schnall MD, Blume J, Bluemke DA, DeAngelis GA, DeBruhl N, Harms S, Heywang- Köbrunner SH, Hylton N, Kuhl CK, Pisano ED, Causer P, Schnitt SJ, Thickman D, Stelling CB, Weatherall PT, Lehman C, Gatsonis CA. Diagnostic architectural and dynamic features at breast MR imaging: multicenter study. Radiology. 2006 Jan;238(1):42-53.
98. Delille JP, Slanetz PJ, Yeh ED, Kopans DB, Halpern EF, Garrido L. Hormone replacement therapy in postmenopausal women: breast tissue perfusion determined with MR imaging-initial observations. Radiology. 2005 Apr;235(1):36-41.
99. Thomassin-Naggara I, Trop I, Chopier J, David J, Lalonde L, Darai E, Rouzier R, Uzan S. Nonmasslike enhancement at breast MR imaging: the added value of mammography and US for lesion categorization. Radiology. 2011 Oct; 261(1):69-79.
100. Rietjens M, Villa G, Toesca A, Rizzo S, Raimondi S, Rossetto F, Sangalli C, De Lorenzi F, Manconi A, Matthes AGZ, Chahuan B, Brenelli F, Bellomi M, Petit JY. Appropriate use of magnetic

resonance imaging and ultrasound to detect early silicone gel breast implant rupture in postmastectomy reconstruction. Plast Reconstr Surg. 2014 Jul;134(1):13e-20e.
101. Wong, T., Lo, L.W., Fung, P.Y.E. et al. Magnetic resonance imaging of breast augmentation: a pictorial review. Insights Imaging 7, 399-410 (2016).
102. Lévy L. IRM et implants mammaires, Imagerie de la femme, December 2008, Pages 236243.
103. Stöblen F, Rezai M, Kümmel S. Imaging in patients with breast implants-results of the First International Breast (Implant) Conference 2009. Insights Imaging. 2010 May;1(2):93-97.
104. Juanpere S, Perez E, Huc O, Motos N, Pont J, Pedraza S. Imaging of breast implants-a pictorial review. Insights Imaging. 2011 Dec;2(6):653-670.
105. Middleton MS. MR evaluation of breast implants. Radiol Clin North Am. 2014 May;52(3):591-608.
106. Safvi A. Linguine sign. Radiology 2000; 216:838-839.
107. Yang N, Muradali D. The augmented breast: a pictorial review of the abnormal and unusual. AJR Am J Roentgenol. 2011 Apr;196(4):W451-60.
108. Seiler SJ, Sharma PB, Hayes JC, Ganti R, Mootz AR, Eads ED, Teotia SS, Evans WP. Multimodality Imaging-based Evaluation of Single-Lumen Silicone Breast Implants for Rupture. Radiographics. 2017 Mar-Apr;37(2):366-382.
109. Soo MS, Kornguth PJ, Walsh R, Elenberger C, Georgiade GS, DeLong D, Spritzer CE. Intracapsular implant rupture: MR findings of incomplete shell collapse. J Magn Reson Imaging. 1997 Jul-Aug;7(4):724-30.
110. Juanpere S, Perez E, Huc O, Motos N, Pont J, Pedraza S. Imaging of breast implants-a pictorial review. Insights Imaging. 2011 Dec;2(6):653-670.
111. Peng HL, Wu CC, Choi WM, Hui MS, Lu TN, Chen LK. Breast cancer detection using magnetic resonance imaging in breasts injected with liquid silicone. Plast Reconstr Surg 1999; 104:2116-2120.
112. Wang J, Shih TT, Chang KJ, Li YW. Silicone migration from silicone-injected breasts: magnetic resonance images. Ann Plast Surg 2002; 48:617-621.
113. Scaranelo AM, Marques AF, Smialowski EB, Lederman HM. Evaluation of the rupture of silicone breast implants by mammography, ultrasonography and magnetic resonance imaging in asymptomatic patients: correlation with surgical findings. Sao Paulo Med J 2004; 122:41-47.
114. Van den Bosch MA, Guit GL, van Waes PF. [Concealed local recurrence after breastconserving treatment]. Ned Tijdschr Geneeskd 2002; 146:1959-1960;
115. Costa SD, Souchon R, Scharl A. [Ipsilateral breast tumor recurrence after conservative breast cancer surgery - diagnosis and therapy]. Zentralbl Gynakol 2004; 126:244-251

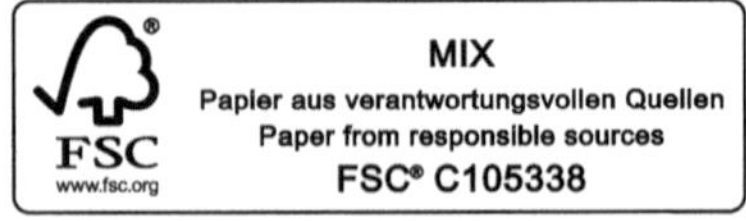

Printed by Books on Demand GmbH, Norderstedt / Germany